THE 3 APPLE A DAY GI DIET

THE 3 APPLE A DAY GI DIET

THE AMAZING SUPERFOOD FOR FAST-TRACK WEIGHT LOSS

TAMMI FLYNN, MS, RD
with Jeanne Drury

HARPER thorsons

HarperThorsons
An imprint of HarperCollins*Publishers*
77–85 Fulham Palace Road,
Hammersmith, London W6 8JB

The website address is: www.thorsonselement.com

and Harper*Thorsons* are trademarks of
HarperCollins*Publishers* Ltd

First self-published in the US in 2003 as *The 3-Apple-a-Day Plan: Your Foundation for Permanent Fat Loss*

This edition published by HarperThorsons 2005

1

A catalogue record of this book is
available from the British Library

ISBN 9780007808458

Printed and bound in Great Britain by
Clays Ltd, St Ives plc

This book is dedicated to my sisters, Tia and Teri, as well as to those of you who are seeking balance and control over food and exercise issues. Finding the path of health that allows you to enjoy the process of eating healthily and exercising will provide you with a sense of well-being and peace—in mind, body, and spirit.

All the best,

Tammi

CONTENTS

ACKNOWLEDGEMENTS

My heartfelt thanks to my friends and family, who have supported me during my book-writing adventure. Cathy Covey, who gave me a copy of *Self-Publishing Manual*, has kept me focused and encouraged through it all.

Others who have helped to ensure accuracy, thoroughness, and creativity throughout the book include Jenny Hymer; Jacki Thomas; Blair McHaney; Chris Lyons; Alice Thompson; Jan Vetter and her daughter Emma; my editor, Jeanne Drury; and designer Ken Trimpe (pulling the all-nighters in the previous edition!).

I especially thank my husband, Dan, who allowed me quiet time and took our three boys to the lake over the weekends. He's truly my best friend and partner, always providing the support and encouragement I need, whatever the endeavour may be.

Finally, many, many thanks to all of you who shared your photos, personal stories, quotes, and wonderful recipes. You made *The 3-Apple-a-Day GI Diet* a success.

Thank you all!

Just knowing what to do is not enough. You need confidence, motivation, and a plan to make permanent changes.

—Anonymous

GETTING STARTED

How much do you want to know?

1. Ready to start the plan today? Go to Quick Start on page 117.
2. Want to learn just the basics? Read only the Key Points at the end of parts I–V (pp. 19, 35, 78, and 88).
3. Want to know the science behind the plan? Read this book from cover to cover.

Ideas to jump-start your motivation

- Take pictures of yourself in a swimsuit (two-piece), front and back, and decide if you want to make a change.
- Train for a marathon.
- Take your doctor's advice to shape up.
- Train to climb Mt Everest.
- Create a get-fit contest in your office.
- Train like an athlete.
- Enrol your family in a "Fit Family Group" and get healthy together.

- Buy an expensive swimsuit in a smaller size and plan a trip to Hawaii.
- Go to your twentieth high-school reunion and check out an old flame or, better yet, the prom queen who snubbed you because you used to be fat!

INTRODUCTION

The 3-Apple-a-Day GI Diet is not about eating apples because they are healthy, even though it's a proven fact that they are. It's about shedding unhealthy fat layers, building strength, keeping lean muscle, and transforming yourself—body and mind—into a fit, self-confident, full-of-life person.

The plan came about by accident as part of the "Get-Lean" Diet I designed for a fitness contest at our gym. In an effort to include more fibre in the diet, in the form of fruits and vegetables, I added an apple before each meal. The results were absolutely astonishing! Who would have guessed that 346 people would lose 6,000 pounds of fat in 12 weeks? Since then, the "accident" has been repeated countless times all over America—with the same amazing fat-loss and body-sculpting results. Read some of the personal success stories in Part V.

If you're tired of diets, pills, and gimmicks and tired of being a human rubbish bin for all kinds of "convenience" foods (which are insidiously turning us into the fattest, unhealthiest people on earth) start the 3-Apple-a-Day GI Diet today for good health, good nutrition, and *permanent fat loss*.

One more thing—be prepared to look and feel fabulous!

How and why it works

The 3-Apple-a-Day GI Diet offers a variety of meals and over 100 recipes custom designed to feed your muscle, not your fat. Each meal is calculated to provide your body with a balance of lean (low-fat) proteins, low-GI (based on the Glycaemic Index), high-fibre carbohydrates, and essential fats. This balance will keep your blood sugar and insulin levels stable, which is necessary for your body to get into a "fat-burning" mode. This balance also helps control your appetite, so you are less tempted by unhealthy foods. The recommended intake of calories, protein, carbohydrates, and fat is based on your current weight so you can maintain lean muscle tissue while shedding the fat.

The 3-Apple-a-Day GI Diet with its moderately high protein level is similar to some of the popular high-protein diets—at first glance. Protein provides calories that do not raise blood sugar, stabilizes blood sugar levels when eaten with carbohydrates, and provides necessary building blocks for maintaining muscle tissue.

Why this diet is different

This plan differs from those popular high-protein diets in two major ways:

1. The focus of the 3-Apple-a-Day GI Diet is not on weight loss alone but primarily fat loss and muscle retention. Many popular diets are based strictly on weight loss, regardless of whether the weight loss is from muscle tissue or fat. When muscle tissue is lost, our metabolism decreases, making it difficult to maintain permanent weight loss.

2. Other high-protein diets are very low in carbohydrates and high in fat, which induces ketosis (a high accumulation of ketones; see Chapter 7 for more on ketosis). People do lose weight quickly with these plans, but, again, they may lose valuable muscle tissue, making it more difficult to keep the weight off. With low carbohydrate consumption comes some unpleasant side-effects, too, such as constipation (due to lack of fibre or bulking carbohydrates), low energy or fatigue during exercise, not to mention mental confusion and moodiness. As if we weren't moody enough already!

   In my professional experience, consuming a diet too low in carbohydrates and/or eating in such a way as to induce ketosis is not an optimum way to retain muscle tissue and achieve permanent fat loss. The key to healthy carbohydrate intake is to consume enough for normal bodily functions (bowel elimination, fuel for the brain and red blood cells), but not in excess.

In the following chapters, you'll find out how, by consuming the right combinations of proteins, carbohydrates, fats, and fibre, you can be successful at permanent fat loss. You'll also find out why thousands of successful "losers" call the 3-Apple-a-Day GI Diet the "terminator" of all diets!

PART I

THE 3 APPLE A DAY GI DIET

CHAPTER 1

The Creation of the 3-Apple-a-Day GI Diet

The beginning

It all started when the American Cancer Society's daily recommendation of five to nine daily servings of fruits and vegetables (in general, a serving is 4 ounces raw or 2 ounces cooked) was proving difficult for one of my personal training clients. She was adamant about getting in her daily requirements but was struggling because she was extremely busy and travelled often. I asked her what her favorite fruit was, and she said apples.

Perfect, I thought. Apples are full of important nutrients, have lots of fibre, taste delicious, and, most important for her, travel well. I suggested she eat an apple before each major meal (breakfast, lunch, and dinner) to see if that would solve her problem.

Amazing results in just seven days

Just one week later, she came back to have her body composition retested saying that since she'd been eating three apples a day, she felt her body had actually changed. She was excited because she hadn't noted any changes for several months.

So we measured, and sure enough, she had lost 1 per cent body fat in one week! Now, a 1 per cent body fat loss (1.5 pounds of fat) in one week is difficult to accomplish in a fit person—and she was already lean at 16 per cent body fat.

"Wow," I said. "Have you been running more?"

She said the only thing she had done differently was to add apples to her meal plan (which actually increased her caloric intake!).

At this point, I was cautiously optimistic. I decided to try this idea on others to see if the results could be duplicated. When Gold's Gym of Wenatchee held its 12-week Get-in-Shape Contest in January 2001, I added apples to the diet (which was then called the "Get Lean" Diet).

The Get-in-Shape Contest

The annual 12-week contest, which I created in 1997, was (and is) a body transformation contest designed to lower body fat while retaining muscle tissue. Although judging is based primarily on visual change from before-and-after pictures, body composition changes are also recorded. As part of the contest, we provided the diet; exercise recommendations; tips on calculating calories, protein, carbohydrates, fat, and water; and other information pertaining to the program.

Apples and the "Get Lean" Diet

The original "Get Lean" Diet was always a balance of low-GI (see Chapter 7 on glycaemic response) carbohydrates, lean proteins, fruits and vegetables, and essential fats—with a calorie distribution of 40 per cent carbohydrates, 40 per cent protein, and 20 per cent fat. On this balanced 12-week fitness contest diet, women averaged a body fat loss of 5 to 7 per cent, and men averaged 7 to 10 per cent loss.

In 2001, when apples were added to the "Get Lean" Diet, Gold's 12-week Get-in-Shape Contest participants experienced record fat losses! Women averaged body fat losses of 7 to 10 per cent, and men averaged losses of 10 to 12 per cent. Not only that, two women broke the "most fat loss" record with 21 per cent body fat loss each! One of those women, who later became a Gold's Gym National winner, lost a whopping 53 pounds of body fat and gained 10 pounds of muscle!

The following year, one male contestant lost 84 pounds of fat and acquired 19 pounds of lean muscle. Another man lost 85 pounds of fat and gained 26 pounds of lean, calorie-burning muscle (see the success stories in Part V).

Remember, these changes were made in just 12 weeks!

What a bunch of (happy) losers!

We were on a roll and truly excited about what we had accomplished. In the 2002 contest, 346 people lost 6,126 pounds of fat. In 2003, 351 people lost 6,453 pounds of fat! In both of those years *five of the ten* Gold's National contest winners hailed from Gold's Gym of little old Wenatchee, Washington!

What's the one thing Wenatchee winners all had in common? You guessed it . . . apples!

But was it *really* the apples?

After the first year of adding apples, even with all our contest successes, I still had reservations about whether apples were actually what helped these contestants lose more body fat than in years past. But adding apples was the only change we had made in the program.

Actually, I had eaten apples for many years when I was dieting for bodybuilding contests, but I never connected eating apples with losing body fat. In fact, I kind of felt like I was cheating when I ate them during my contest dieting phase—because they tasted so good!

It wasn't until I had read some of the contestants' amazing and inspiring personal stories—writing a personal story was a requirement for completion of the contest—that I was finally convinced. There just were too many testimonials naming apples as a major contributor to contestants' success to be a mere coincidence.

The $500,000 Gold's Gym Challenge

I became a true believer, and I was not alone. The entire staff at Gold's Gym in Wenatchee was so strongly convinced that apples were a key to people's weight-loss efforts that we approached the Washington Apple Commission and Gold's Gym Corporate about sponsoring a national contest.

Of course, the folks at corporate headquarters were sceptical at first. But with real numbers, testimonials, and real contestants, they signed on to the idea, and the $500,000 Gold's Gym Challenge was born. At the same time, Gold's Gym Corporate adopted the Washington apple as "the Official Diet Pill of Gold's Gym".

How and why do apples work in fat loss?

> I was never hungry. In fact, I had to retrain myself to eat enough. Never tiring of the three apples per day, I had no cravings for sweets. I believe the sweet Fuji apples helped in this area. I looked forward to having my apple as a snack every

night! I had more energy and was amazed at how steadily I lost weight. I plan to continue using the 3-Apple-a-Day GI Diet to maintain my weight.

—Sandi Anderson, age 53, lost 31 pounds of fat and gained 2 pounds of muscle in 12 weeks

When the Gold's Gym Challenge began, I started getting a lot of questions about apples, mostly about how they work in fat loss and what research I had to back up the claims of significant fat loss from our contestants.

At first, I was unaware of any research studies that linked apples with weight loss—let alone fat loss! I chose apples originally because of their convenience, their sweet, crunchy texture, and their high fibre content (4 to 5 grams per apple). I had found a few studies linking increased fibre intake to weight loss, because increased fibre intake was associated with decreasing hunger and food intake, but none naming apples as the fibre source.

Recently, a Brazilian study of overweight women compared diets that contained three apples per day, three pears per day, or oat cookies, to determine their respective effects on body weight. The results showed that the women who ate either three apples or three pears per day lost significantly more weight than did the oat cookie group. This study is similar to what we found in our Gold's Gym contest.

Apples are one of the only fruits that have high amounts of both soluble and insoluble fibre. The soluble fibre, pectin, helps steady your blood sugar. Researcher Kay-Tee Khaw at Cambridge University says, "Pectin turns into a sticky gel as you digest it, keeping your stomach from absorbing the sugar too quickly." According to a study published in the *Journal of the American College of Nutrition*, pectin eliminates the urge to eat for up to four hours.

Apples, too, are low on the Glycaemic Index (see Chapter 7), at a rating of 38 (compared with sugar at 70 or maltose at 105). Low-GI foods don't spike your blood sugar level, making them an ideal appetizer prior to a main meal or a perfect snack between meals.

In a more general sense, a 12-year Harvard study of 74,000 women, funded by the National Heart, Lung, and Blood Institute, concluded that those who consumed more fruits and vegetables were 26 per cent less likely to become obese than women who ate fewer fruits and vegetables over the same time period.

Also, many studies have shown that apples can help in other aspects of health, such as preventing heart disease, stroke, and cancer and improving lung function and dental health.

The phenomenal increase in fat loss that thousands of Gold's Gym clients experienced when they added apples to their diet plans, along with their personal testimonials naming apples as a key component to their success, is a more compelling reason for controlled studies to be done at the scientific level.

Right now, we'll settle for what works!

Good news for people with Type 2 diabetes

The 3-Apple-a-Day GI Diet is also used by Gold's Gym of Wenatchee in other challenges. One of those, the Type 2 Diabetes Challenge, is a six-month program based on a point system. As with the Get-in-Shape Contest, using the same diet and measuring body fat only, the contestants were required to keep food, beverage, medicine, and exercise journals; to test their blood sugar twice a day and blood pressure once a week; and to have pre- and post-challenge lipid (blood fats) profiles, including cholesterol and triglycerides (see Chapter 10), and an A1C test (a measure used to determine long-term blood sugar control). The participants did not have any kidney dysfunction before starting or after finishing the challenge.

The results from the Type 2 Diabetes Challenge showed that the group that ate at least three apples per day lost an average of 19 pounds of body fat. The group that ate only one to two apples per day lost 11 pounds of body fat. The other group, which ate one or no apple per day, lost only 3 pounds of body fat. Overall, the average A1C reading was reduced from 7.5 at the starting point to under 5 (normal range) at the finish.

Similar results were obtained with our six-month Wellness Challenge. The parameters were similar as far as keeping food, beverage, medicine, and exercise journals plus pre- and post-challenge lipid and glucose panels. Again, we saw a correlation between eating three apples a day and the greatest fat loss and a lowering of total cholesterol (mainly LDLs).

Worried about cholesterol? More good news

Most people who had high blood lipids before following the 3-Apple-a-Day GI Diet experienced dramatic changes in their blood work afterward. Exercise and eating the foods on the plan not only lowered their total cholesterol, LDLs, triglycerides, and blood pressure, but increased their HDLs (good cholesterol).

Here's a great example. Byron, a 40-year-old male, started with an unhealthy cholesterol level of 211 and triglycerides level of 637. In week 11 of the program, his cholesterol fell to an amazing 97 (the low end of the range) and triglycerides to 51 (normal range)! On top of that, his HDLs improved from a low of 25 to a normal level of 35. With astonishment, his doctor asked if he felt OK and suggested they double-check to make sure the readings were accurate. Byron said he hadn't felt this good since high school. And yes, the reading was accurate!

Others around the country also noted improvements in their blood work. Richard from Utah lost 36 pounds and lowered his cholesterol from 218 to 152. More important, his LDLs went from 128 to 86 and his triglycerides from 270 to 61. His HDLs increased from 36 to 49.

Scott from Maine lost 83 pounds and lowered his cholesterol from 243 to 125. His LDLs dropped from 133 to 58, and his triglycerides fell from 220 to 55.

Pete from Florida lost 53 pounds, lowered his cholesterol from 278 to 176, decreased his LDLs from 180 to 116, and his triglycerides from 309 to 58. His HDLs improved from 36 to 48. Pete's doctor told him he was a heartbeat away from a heart attack before he started the 3-Apple-a-Day GI Diet. When his final blood work was done, the doctor couldn't believe the improvements Pete had made in just 12 weeks!

Who can use this plan?

The 3-Apple-a-Day GI Diet is useful for most people. My clients consist of women and men of all ages—ranging from 18 to 80—many of whom have adopted the plan for their entire family. Others, who have heart disease, high blood pressure, thyroid dysfunction, and Type 2 diabetes, are interested in improving their health and reducing their medications.

As mentioned earlier, people with Type 2 diabetes have been very successful using this plan. According to the Centers for Disease Control and Prevention (CDC), there are 17 million Americans with Type 2 diabetes, currently termed the "obese disease". This number has tripled since 1960 and is anticipated to triple again by 2050. By that time, one in three children born in 2000 will have diabetes if people don't start adopting a healthier lifestyle—meaning healthier eating and more exercise. What's even more frightening is that the CDC estimates 70 million Americans are currently overweight, including one out of four children!

And the numbers are rising in the UK, too, as more and more adults and children are becoming overweight or obese.

What exactly do we mean by "overweight"? That's a tricky question. I'll discuss it in the next chapter. The answer may surprise you, and it is one of the things that sets the 3-Apple-a-Day GI Diet apart from any diet you've tried before.

> Always check with your doctor before starting a food program, especially if you have had previous health risks.

CHAPTER 2

Overweight versus Overfat

What's the difference?

Researchers have learned that body fat, instead of weight, is a better predictor of health. High body fat, or "overfat", is associated with conditions such as Type 2 diabetes, heart disease, high blood pressure, insulin resistance, and cancer.

Being overfat is more dangerous to your health than being overweight. Traditionally, being overweight has been defined as weighing more than the healthy weight listed for your age and height in a weight table. But that doesn't account for differences in body composition. For example, athletes are often overweight according to the weight-table standards because of muscle development or large body frame, but they are probably not overfat.

The 3-Apple-a-Day GI Diet was specifically designed and developed for permanent fat loss and muscle retention (keeping lean muscle tissue). This plan was not necessarily designed for weight loss—at least using the traditional method of measure, the scales. Other measuring techniques to determine progress have been highly effective and motivational. These include girth measurements (waist, hip, and thigh), body composition testing, and body mass index, which we'll get into later.

The scales tells you only the partial truth

Weighing yourself on bathroom scales tells you next to nothing about how healthy you really are. Gaining or losing a pound doesn't always mean it's a pound of fat. In fact, small, frequent shifts in weight typically reflect fluid changes in your body. Your body's fluid levels vary depending on the amount of salt you eat, your activity level, and hormonal changes. It seems that many people, mainly women, are controlled by the numbers on the scales. If the number goes up, they're discouraged. If the number goes down, they are motivated and happy. The numbers on the scales do not measure the progress you have made, and they can even be detrimental to your program. *Why not break those barriers and get permanent results without the frustration of the scales?* The following photos show how people with different body types and levels of body fat, and different degrees of lean muscle can weigh the same.

Males 40–49 years old

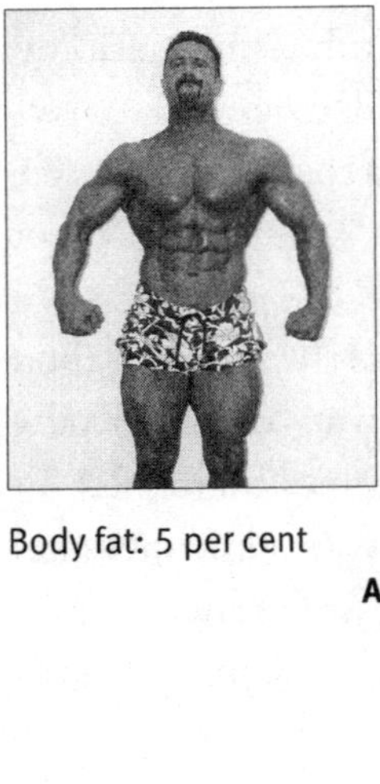

Body fat: 5 per cent

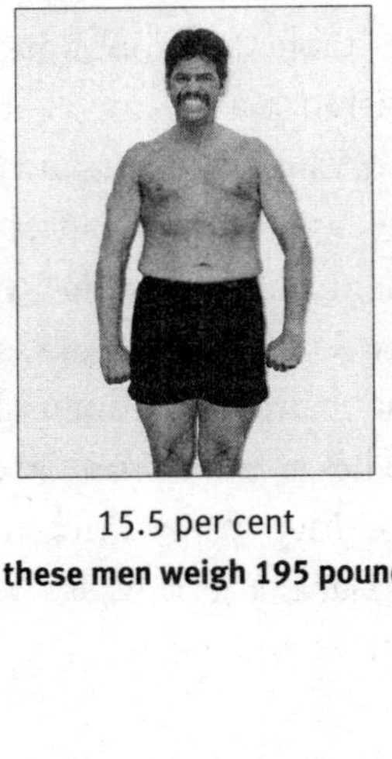

15.5 per cent

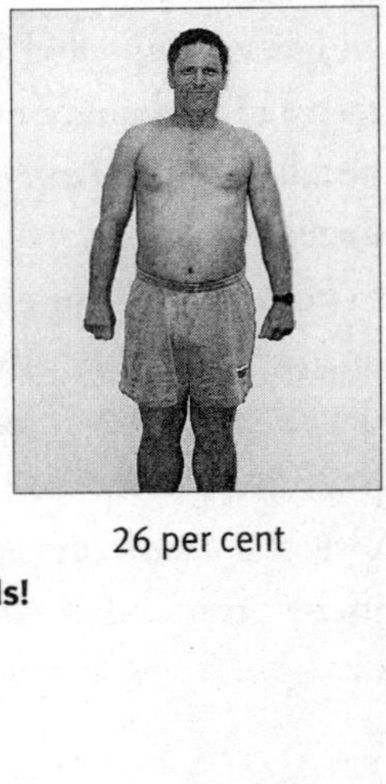

26 per cent

All these men weigh 195 pounds!

Females 30–39 years old

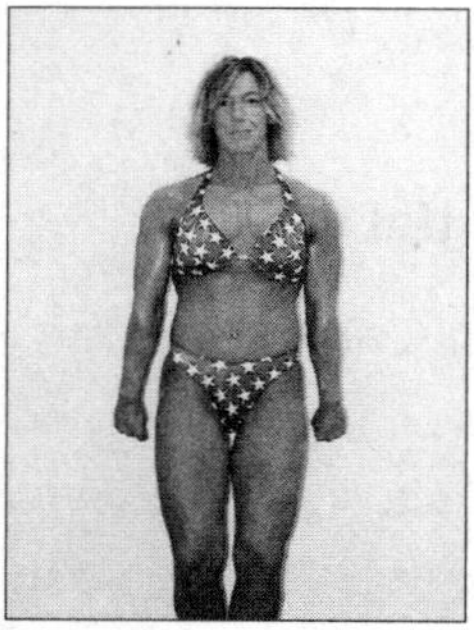

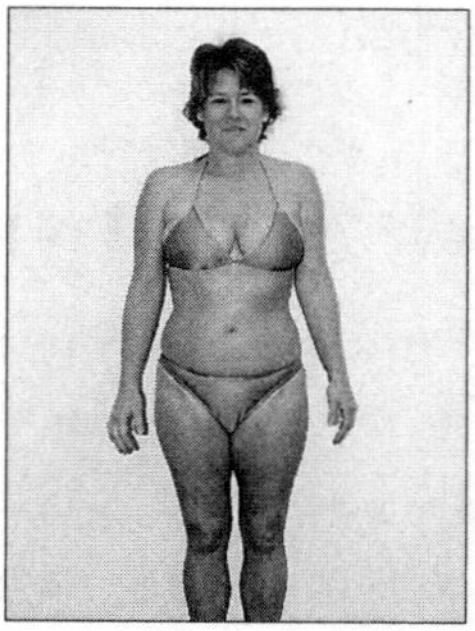

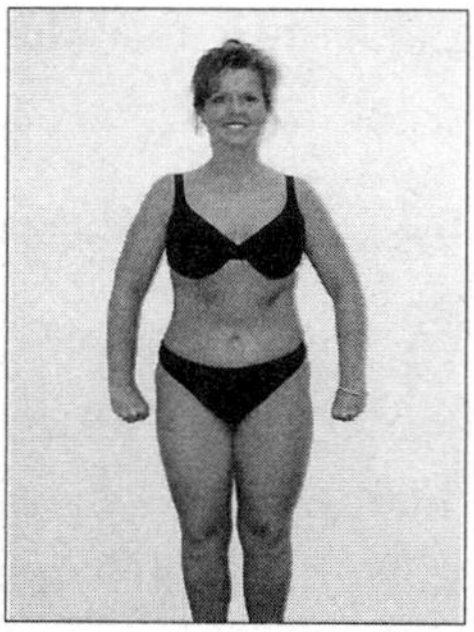

Body fat: 13 per cent 23 per cent 31 per cent

All these women weigh 135 pounds!

Get the picture?

Other methods for measuring

Methods of body-fat measuring that should be done by a trained professional include skinfold measurements, infrared interactance, bioelectrical impedance, and underwater weighing. Other methods, such as girth measurements and body mass index (BMI), can be done at home. A BMI reading is based on your height and weight and is just a gauge for determining health risk. This measurement may not be appropriate for athletes or very active people. The 3-Apple-a-Day GI Diet asks you to chart your girth measurements.

For girth measurements, use a tape measure. Measure the waist at the navel, the hips around the buttocks, and the thighs at their upper part. Every one inch lost from the waist is equal to 4 pounds of body fat (*Muscle and Fitness* magazine, March 2003). Use the chart on page 15 to keep track of your girth measurements in inches as you work the 3-Apple-a-Day GI Diet.

Charting Girth Measurements

	Date	Waist	Hips	Thigh
Start	____	____	____	____
Week 2	____	____	____	____
Week 4	____	____	____	____
Week 6	____	____	____	____
Week 8	____	____	____	____
Week 10	____	____	____	____
Week 12	____	____	____	____
Total change		–____	–____	–____

Calculating Body Mass Index (BMI)

To determine BMI, use the following formula (or use the free calculator at nhlbisupport.com/bmi):

Weight (pounds) ÷ Height (inches)^2 × 703 = BMI

Example: Female, 140 pounds, 5 foot 4 inches
140 ÷ (64" × 64") × 703 = 24

Example: Male, 185 pounds, 5 foot 11 inches
185 ÷ (71" × 71") × 703 = 25.79

If your BMI ranges from 18.5 to 24.9, your weight is not likely to have a major effect on your health. If your BMI is 25 or more, talk to your GP about the 3-Apple-a-Day GI Diet.

Is it time to act?

The health questionnaire on page 16 is a screening tool to help you assess your physical activity and nutrition habits. Whether you find that you're at high risk of becoming overfat or not, answering the questions may increase your awareness about your current habits. If you have decided that you could stand some

Is your health at risk?

- Do you eat at *least* five servings of fruits and vegetables per day?
- Are you physically active at least 30 minutes per day, seven days per week?
- Do you eat fewer than three deep-fried foods per week?
- Is your waist measurement under 35 inches for a female? Under 40 inches for a male?
- Is your BMI under 25?
- Do you consider yourself at a healthy body fat level?
- Does your family history show healthy body weights without obesity?

If you can answer yes to most of these questions, you're probably not at high risk of developing overfat-related diseases. If you answered no to at least three of the questions, your chances are greater for developing overfat-related diseases.

This is not a medically proven questionnaire to determine the risk of becoming overfat. It is used exclusively as a screening technique for increasing health awareness.

improvement, try simply changing one of your undesirable food or activity habits instead of focusing on the scales. Use *The 3-Apple-a-Day GI Diet* for guidance. You will be amazed at how easily the fat will come off when you make even small changes, such as eating an apple before every meal.

In the next chapter, we'll look at other factors that determine if you'll become overfat, and we'll see how the 3-Apple-a-Day GI Diet can make a big difference.

CHAPTER 3

Genetics and Obesity

Were we born to be fat?

Genetics play a role in your body type and how you store fat. Yet other factors greatly influence your risk of being fat or overfat—factors that you can change or prevent.

The big fat facts of life

Fact one: we can't always blame our parents. Yes, our genes affect the rate at which our body accumulates fat and where the fat is stored. And, yes, a family history of obesity does increase our chances of becoming obese (overfat) by about 30 per cent, and of course our family affected our eating habits and activity levels when we were children. But we have 70 per cent control over how healthy and fit we are as adults—what we do to take control is up to us.

Fact two: No matter who we are, we all have an unlimited potential to make new fat cells, which means we all risk obesity and obesity-related diseases if we continue to overeat and under-exercise.

So now's the time to start making changes. The thousands of people who have followed the 3-Apple-a-Day GI Diet have come from a variety of backgrounds. Most everyone who stuck with the plan has seen great results.

The difference between boys and girls

Have you ever wondered why men seem to lose weight at the drop of a hat and women seem to have more of a struggle? Or why building muscle seems to come naturally to guys but takes longer for us gals? Does "you are what you eat" ring a bell?

In my 20 years of experience in the health and fitness industry, I have observed that men and women have different preferences, which may influence how they lose body fat. When it comes to food preferences, for example, men tend to choose protein over carbohydrates. In terms of exercise, they go for the weight training every time—with as little cardiovascular training as possible.

My women clients, on the other hand, prefer carbohydrates over protein, and they choose walking for weight loss (cardiovascular training) instead of weight training.

Are you connecting the dots?

Muscle, fat, and metabolism

Because of their higher muscle mass, men tend to burn 10 to 20 per cent more calories than do women (who have higher levels of body fat). Think about this: 1 pound of muscle tissue burns 40 to 60 calories per day whereas 1 pound of fat tissue burns a measly 2 calories per day. No wonder these guys lose weight so easily. Their higher muscle mass endows them with a higher metabolic rate. But ladies, you can change all that by adding some muscle mass through weight training!

Use it or lose it!

As you age, if you do not use your muscles, you'll lose them. The muscle tissue shrinks, resulting in lower metabolism and an inability to burn calories. Starting around age 25, you lose about 1 per cent of muscle every year, which results in a reduction of metabolism. So let's do the maths.

By the age of 35, you will have lost approximately 5 pounds of muscle. For each pound of muscle lost, you lose the ability to burn 40 to 60 calories per day. So 5 pounds of muscle times 40 to 60 calories per day equals 200 to 300 calories less that your body is able to burn per day. By the age of 50, you may have lost 25 pounds of muscle, reducing your calorie-burning ability by 1,000

Key Points from Part I

- Try to see the big picture. Having a balanced eating and exercise plan will help you become a fit, self-confident, full-of-life person.
- The 3-Apple-a-Day GI Diet is a balance of lean proteins, low-GI and high-fibre carbohydrates, and essential fats.
- Eat three apples per day, one before each major meal.
- Apples are full of fibre—4 to 5 grams each—and fibre has been shown to be effective in weight loss.
- Being overfat, not just overweight, brings a higher risk of obesity-related diseases.
- Avoid the scales for measuring your fitness progress. Use the tape measure instead.
- Genetics has only a small influence on becoming overfat. You have 70 per cent control.
- Muscle tissue burns more calories than does fat tissue.
- Weight training builds muscle tissue.

calories. You may begin to notice that you eat less, but you are getting fatter. Although this may be somewhat exaggerated, I think you get the point.

But all is not lost. Weight training increases muscle mass, which increases your ability to burn calories. It's possible to minimize, even reverse, some of the damage from inactivity—if you start now!

If your goal is permanent fat loss, weight training is the answer, and it is a vital part of the 3-Apple-a-Day GI Diet (see Part IV on exercise).

PART II

MENTAL PREPARATION

CHAPTER 4

You Have the Power!

If your eating habits have been less than healthy, you have the power to make the change! Every step you take to improve your health will get you closer to adding life into your years. The foods you choose, along with your activity level, will determine whether you become fat or not. The most notable causes of being overfat or obese are lack of proper diet and lack of physical activity. Thank goodness these are things you can change. If you can visualize it, you can become it!

> Being an obese, out-of-control Type 2 diabetic, I talked with my doctor, who said he could no longer help me, I had to help myself. Then I heard the words "train like an athlete". So I started practising being an athlete—started a food and exercise journal, joined the gym, bought athletic clothes so I could look like an athlete, and after work and days off I would change into my athletic clothes to feel like an athlete. So who cares if I looked like the Pillsbury Doughboy®? In my mind I was an athlete.
>
> **—Donald Housden, age 55, lost 33 pounds, and is now an athlete**

Getting and staying motivated

How do you get motivated and stay motivated? Motivation comes from within. *Webster's Dictionary* defines "motivation" as "a mental force to induce an act or purpose". "Inspiration" is any influence that inspires thought or action. What inspires you?

I have found that my clients are inspired by money, family, and other people's successes. In the beginning, you may be motivated to win (through a bet) or to look like someone else (if they can do it, so can I), or you may believe that if you can make a change it will help inspire your family to change. But what will really keep you progressing towards your goal is how good you'll feel as the changes add up.

Some people are naturally self-motivated and others need a little extra help from outside influences. Here are a few ideas that may inspire you to get started:

- Try a walkathon.
- Train for a marathon.
- Shape up for your class reunion.
- Work out with your significant other.
- Decide to improve your family's eating habits.
- Aim to fit into your smallest clothes size.
- Read the success stories in Part V.

> **TIP:** Find something or someone that inspires you. Health clubs can be inspirational because you're surrounded by people with a common interest—getting healthy!

Are timelines a good thing?

Does focusing on a short period of time, such as 12 weeks instead of a lifetime, prove unsuccessful for permanent fat loss? It all depends on whether you are enjoying the experience of getting fit or struggling throughout the entire process. You may be highly motivated when you first start a new diet or exercise program, but maybe your motivation dissipates over time if you cannot see or feel results.

Most people who start the 3-Apple-a-Day GI Diet adjust over the first few weeks and are excited by how good they feel. For some, it's more difficult, especially if they've never exercised or been aware of their eating habits. On the other hand, if they finish the 12 weeks, they are thrilled with their progress. And more important, most of them maintain their results.

Twelve weeks will pass by anyway, so why not do something during that time that will make a difference in how you look and feel? Think of 12 weeks as just the beginning of a lifetime of healthy behaviours.

> **TIP:** Set small, realistic, short-term goals that will lead you to your major goal. If you bite off more than you can chew, it can be overwhelming!

CHAPTER 5

The Importance of Setting Goals

Health versus fitness

What is your goal in following the 3-Apple-a-Day GI Diet? Do you want to improve your health or improve your fitness? This is an important question because the answer helps determine what goals to set. You can improve your health by making simple or major changes such as adding or increasing activity, improving diet, quitting smoking, reducing stress, getting adequate rest, and laughing.

Yes, laughing. According to William Fry, MD, professor at Stanford University, who has conducted 50 years of laughter research, laughter conditions the heart muscle, exercises the lungs, works all the abdominal thoracic muscles, boosts the immune system, and even increases adrenaline and blood flow to the brain. Humour can add years to your life! Many of these changes will show up in improved mental health status but not necessarily as a noticeable physical change.

Fitness improvements may take more effort. But the resulting change in body fat, increased muscle tissue, cardiovascular and respiratory efficiency, and improved mental alertness will all be worth the extra sweat!

That said, fitness goals require fitness-oriented strategies, including a regular exercise routine, a well-balanced meal plan, adequate rest, and a plan of action. The 3-Apple-a-Day GI Diet is designed for fitness-oriented people, but most people can use this plan for health improvements, too.

Determining your goals

Do you want to run to your goal or walk? In other words, do you want to achieve your goal quickly or make gradual changes? Goals need to be set according to what you are planning to accomplish. The 3-Apple-a-Day GI Diet was designed for people who want to lose body fat and keep their muscle tissue. The following examples may give you some ideas for setting goals:

1. Although weight loss should not be the primary focus, most health experts agree that 1 or 2 pounds of weight loss per week is safe and healthy. Rapid and extreme weight loss can also result in muscle loss, which is often associated with low-calorie meal plans.

> **TIP:** Make your goals specific and measurable so you'll know what you've achieved.

2. Reducing your clothes size is a measurable goal. Get out your smallest-size clothes so they're visible. If you can see it, you can achieve it!
3. Waist, hip, and thigh reduction—measure those areas and try to lose one inch per month in your "problem" area (waist or hips).

4. Lower your cholesterol, blood pressure, or blood sugar by starting a regular exercise routine.
5. Increase your daily energy by improving your eating exercise and habits. You can measure your progress by keeping a food and exercise journal (see the section on journaling later in this chapter).
6. Gain strength or increase lean muscle tissue through weight training. Improvements can be measured by increased weights lifted or body composition testing.
7. Commit to eating breakfast every day.
8. Switch the nightly food binge to fruits, vegetables, or lean proteins only.
9. Reduce body fat to the healthy range—women 17 to 24 per cent, men 14 to 20 per cent.
10. Exercise for 20 minutes during your lunch hour every day.

The list can go on. It may take several small goals to achieve your results. I call these "mini-goals".

Put it in writing

A great way to launch a new health-and-fitness regime is to commit yourself to it on paper. That's what the 3-Apple-a-Day Personal Contract is all about.

When filling out your contract, first start by determining what you'd really like to achieve—your ultimate goal. All mini-goals will be set to lead to your main objective. Think of it as walking up stairs—eventually you reach the top. How long it takes will depend on what your ultimate goal is. Take some time to think realistically about your goals. If you decide you want to lose 50 pounds but you've never been that light, then this type of goal may not be realistic in a short time frame. An example of the contract is on the next page.

Tammi's Personal Contract

I, *Tammi Flynn,* plan to accomplish my ultimate goal of *competing in a mini-triathlon.* To reach this goal, I have established several mini-goals, which are as follows: 1. *Continue the 3-Apple-a-Day GI Diet.* 2. *Start swimming on Mondays, Wednesdays, and Fridays at 6 A.M.* 3. *Increase my biking to four days per week, 45 minutes each.* I am beginning my journey on *Monday, July 5,* to reach my ultimate goal by *September 18.* I will continue to move forward and redefine my goals. My motivation level is *extremely high.* As I reach each of my mini-goals, I will reward myself weekly by *getting a massage.*

Signed by: *Tammi Flynn*

Date: *July 1.*

Support person: *husband, Dan*

The 3-Apple-a-Day GI Diet Personal Contract

I, ____________________, plan to accomplish my ultimate goal of ____________________________. To reach this goal, I have established several mini-goals, which are as follows: 1. ____________________. 2. ____________________________. 3. ____________________.
I am beginning my journey on this date: ____________________.
I would like to reach my ultimate goal by this date: ______________.
If I don't make this date, I will continue to move forward and redefine my goals. My motivation level is [circle one] high very high extremely high. As I reach each of my mini-goals, I will reward myself by ____.

Signed by: ______________________________

Date: ______________________________

Support person:* ______________________________

**Check in with this person every two weeks and let him or her know how you are doing.*

Find someone to lean on

The Personal Contract has a place for the name of a support person. This person should not only cheer you on but also hold you accountable to your contract for as long as you want him or her to. My husband, Dan, is my support person, and he takes care of the kids in the mornings so I can go swimming. He also checks my training journal each week.

Give yourself a treat

Finally, think about how you will reward yourself for reaching your goals. Just make sure your reward isn't an unhealthy choice and a step in the wrong direction. Some positive rewards include a massage (my favourite!), a manicure, or a good book. One of my clients hires a babysitter every Friday afternoon for two hours so she can do whatever she wants. It's usually shopping!

Journaling prevents "amnesia"

Keeping a food and exercise journal is a key way to stick with your plan. Writing down an accurate record of your intake of food and beverages daily and recording the calories, protein, fat, carbohydrates, and fibre will help you become more aware of what is in the foods you eat.

Writing it down will also hold you accountable for what you have been eating or drinking. Although you may have good intentions, what you intend and what you actually do may be two different things. I call this "amnesia". An exercise journal works the same way. You'll know if you are making progress by keeping records of where you were when you started. In the Appendix, you'll find a sample form for keeping a food and beverage record (page 219).

Tips from Past Contest Winners at Gold's Gym

1. Keep a food and exercise journal. This keeps you accountable and on track.
2. Focus on a specific goal. **Visualize your end result.** Keep reminding yourself that you are committed to achieving that goal.
3. Plan, prepare, and commit.

   Plan what you want to accomplish (goal), how long it will take you (time line), and how you can accomplish your goal (specific program).

   Prepare—know what you'll be eating and when you'll be exercising daily. Prepare meals ahead of time and plan your workout before you get to the gym.

   Commit—make a contract with yourself, spouse, children, or trainer to accomplish your goals. Again, be specific and use this contract to hold yourself accountable.

If you fail to plan, you plan to fail. *—Nancy Vanhoven, group fitness instructor, Gold's Gym of Wenatchee, Washington*

Don't kid yourself

A frustrated client e-mailed me saying she had been following the plan but wasn't making any progress. I asked if she was writing anything down. She wasn't. I asked her to keep a journal and send it to me after a few days so I could see where she might be struggling. No wonder she hadn't made progress! Her journal indicated that she ate almost everything out of a box or a container! Except for eating two apples per day, she wasn't following the plan at all. In addition, she hadn't changed her exercise program (walking) for over a year. I made some suggestions in order to accommodate her busy schedule (the reason for her dependence on convenience foods) and food preferences. A few weeks later, she e-mailed back to say, happily I might add, that she had finally started seeing some results.

Again, your intentions may be good, but writing it down is the only way to outsmart your biased and forgetful mind!

Breaking barriers and excuses, excuses, excuses!

Why is it that when we start an exercise or food program we often don't follow through (as in "it seemed like a good idea at the time")? There are a few legitimate reasons that may be out of your control that can inhibit you from reaching your goals—such as illness or certain disabilities. But mostly, barriers are excuses that keep you in your comfort zone—or rather, out of your discomfort zone! Changing eating and exercise habits may be one of the most difficult challenges you'll experience. But remember, the rewards you'll gain far outweigh those initial struggles.

Here are some of the common controllable barriers that factor into changing your lifestyle habits:

- *Not enough time to exercise*. Exercise needs to be a priority just like brushing your teeth!
- *Too intimidated to go to the gym because you're out of shape*. Start walking or working out at home with exercise videos. But remember that a good gym can offer professional help to guide you to your goals.
- *The belief that you need a diet very low in calories in order to lose weight*. Eating too few calories is a sure way to lose valuable muscle tissue. Women need at least 1,200 calories per day, and men need at least 1,800.
- *Environment*. You're surrounded by a feasting society. Fast foods and quick-food markets are loaded with high-fat, high-sugar, nutrient-light temptations. When you plan ahead and prepare your meals yourself, the temptations will become less, and you will not have to rely on willpower.

- *No energy or too tired.* The first thing many people notice when they start following the 3-Apple-a-Day GI Diet is that they have more energy. Get started, you'll see!

Beware of emotional triggers—They make you eat!

Have you ever been sad and sat down with a tub of ice cream smothered in chocolate and just kept eating it? Or been stressed out and stuffed a whole bag of crisps (family size!) in your face? Or just felt bored and wandered through your kitchen "searching" for something interesting to eat and discovered (and ate) your kid's leftover Halloween candy? Or felt the "winding down" of a busy day and needed a little pick-me-up from food?

This is emotional eating. There are several emotional triggers—anger, stress/anxiety, PMS, boredom, and sadness—that cause us to eat. And we usually don't choose healthy snacks in this state of mind. Instead, we choose "comfort foods" that temporarily fill the void. Often, not only do we consume way too much of these foods but we repeat this type of eating way too often, all of which leads to weight gain and low self-esteem.

How to break the cycle

Breaking the cycle of emotional eating may take some effort. But you can do it! When you feel one or more of the emotional triggers come on, resist the urge for five minutes. Ask yourself if you are truly hungry or are just feeling emotional? Often just waiting a couple of minutes will be sufficient to overcome the urge. If waiting doesn't work and you are still feeling emotional, try diverting yourself. Go outside for some fresh air, take a walk, turn on some upbeat music, or call a supportive friend.

If you do decide to eat, choose a healthy snack. Dip some unsalted pretzels in yogurt or spread apple slices with peanut butter. Or treat yourself to some low-fat popcorn and a diet beverage. And don't turn on the television! Huh? That's right! Watching TV could actually cause you to "unconsciously" eat more.

I definitely have times of emotional overeating—where do you think the examples came from? What I have found to work, besides avoiding unhealthy snacks, is having an established eating plan. If you follow the 3-Apple-a-Day GI Diet, as I do, you should be able to keep your appetite under control and lessen those unhealthy food temptations.

Hunger versus appetite

Blair McHaney, co-owner of Gold's Gym, Wenatchee, Washington, suggests this visual: "Think of appetite as a sleeping lion. If you keep him fed, he will purr and sleep. If you starve him, he will attack." The lion is your appetite. If you aren't prepared with food on hand, your appetite may attack and you'll be relying on your willpower. That's doing it the hard way for sure.

It's a lot easier to shop for healthy foods in the supermarket if you are not hungry as a lion going in. Not only that, if you don't go in hungry, you'll be less likely to buy unhealthy items. It's much easier to decide not to buy junk food than it is to resist it once you've taken it home. Keep your home environment "safe" and junk-food free to avoid temptation.

Last but not least, eat breakfast! You'll be less likely to eat a donut at work if you've already eaten at home.

> **TIP:** Take apples with you everywhere you go.

Key Points of Part II

- If you can visualize what you want to become, it will happen.
- Keep a food and beverage journal.
- Set your ultimate goal. Make sure it's realistic and measurable.
- Set measurable mini-goals to help you reach your ultimate goal.
- Find some inspiration to motivate you.
- Break the barriers that prevent you from reaching your goal.
- Prepare and plan so willpower won't be an issue.

PART III

GOOD NUTRITION

CHAPTER 6

The Truth about Nutrition, Diet, and Fat Loss

Mass confusion

There are simply too many diet books, versions of food pyramids, and guidelines and too much other nutritional advice on the market today. Each source would have you believe theirs is *the one*. Much of the information is conflicting. Should you eat a low-fat, high-carbohydrate diet? Or a low-carbohydrate, high-fat diet? Should you eat high-protein, high-fat? How about the no-dairy, no-wheat, no-fat, no-meat (and no flavour) diet? Just kidding!

Amid the cacophony of opinions, there is one thing that most experts do agree on. Most people are overfat because they don't eat enough fruits and vegetables and they don't engage in regular physical activity. It's as simple as that.

The low-calorie weight-loss trap

> I had to laugh when I heard the phrase "skinny fat person", and that's when it hit me. That's what I have ended up being every time I went on a diet because all that I did was stop eating and didn't have a real exercise program. Then my weight always ended up coming back even heavier than I was to begin with!
>
> **—Jim Barker, age 51, lost 43.5 pounds of body fat and gained 0.5 pound of muscle**

Many of the popular programs these days are based strictly on weight loss. Losing weight can be beneficial for many reasons aside from appearance—*but only if you can maintain your current muscle mass*.

Some of these plans are downright harmful, especially if permanent fat loss is your goal. For example, the diets based on very low calories are the biggest trap of all. They are seductive in that they offer quick results. But in the long term they are disastrous. Ultra-low-calorie diets are the cause of yo-yo dieting, which lowers your metabolism incrementally over time until it's almost impossible to lose weight.

Research from the University of California has shown that crash diets—of fewer than 1,000 calories a day—slow metabolism down by as much as 45 per cent!

These diets fly in the face of what is now common knowledge: To raise your metabolism, you have to *eat more healthy foods, not eat less!* Eating less lowers your metabolism by stripping away your muscle tissue. It is the direct cause of the dieting plateaus that are so hard to overcome. It's likely you'll become a "skinny fat person" if you follow a low-calorie eating program.

"But," you reason, "if I eat more I'll just gain weight."

Not if you eat healthy foods and exercise you won't. If you consume small, nutritionally balanced, low-GI meals, at regular intervals throughout the day, your metabolism will be revved up all day long.

In other words, you need the 3-Apple-a-Day GI Diet.

Why I wrote this book

I'm not a diet guru on the talk show circuit. I'm not selling supplements or magic weight-loss powders. What I am is a registered dietitian, a bodybuilder, and a group training instructor with 20 years of experience in helping my clients lose fat, get fit—and stay fit.

My purpose in writing this book is to use my knowledge of nutrition, diet, and exercise to guide you to *permanent fat loss and muscle retention* without diet pills, supplements, or gimmicks. I would also like to clear the air of the confusion and disinformation associated with nutrition and weight loss.

The 3-Apple-a-Day GI Diet draws on all food groups in balanced proportions to help your metabolism do its job. It features apples because of their convenience, low glycaemic rating, and high fibre content—the latter two of which are extremely important in fat loss.

The control you need to succeed

The 3-Apple-a-Day GI Diet will give you the control you must have over your appetite in order to achieve your weight loss goals. You can achieve this control by balancing carbohydrates, proteins, and essential fats.

The plan is for people who want to make the most out of their lives, without perpetually looking for the one and only "next best diet". Most important, this plan when combined with an exercise program, has been successful in helping people achieve *permanent* fat loss.

Nutrient recommendations

The next few chapters explain how the different elements in your diet can make you healthier or make you sick. Throughout I refer to the DRIs. These are the US Institute of Medicine's Food and Nutrition Board Dietary Reference Intakes (DRIs). They provide guidance on how much of each nutrient is needed in a healthy diet. These chapters will help you understand the importance of the major nutrients in your diet so that you can maximize your fat-loss efforts while getting lasting energy from the foods you eat. They will also make sense of the recommendations in the 3-Apple-a-Day GI Diet.

CHAPTER 7

Carbohydrates—Good Food for Your Brain

The misunderstood nutrient

I feel good when I think of carbohydrates, because I know they provide the right kind of fuel for my brain cells. Unfortunately, many people shun them as if they were the plague. The fact is, carbohydrates have gotten a bad rap recently for weight-loss efforts, just like fat has in years past.

What's more (and what dieters aren't aware of), the types of carbohydrates you choose can affect your fat-loss progress to a *very high degree*. So let's set the record straight with the facts on carbohydrates.

Diet fads seem to come in cycles. Remember when protein was the enemy and carbohydrates were the answer? Now the opposite philosophy is the new big thing. Yet with new findings about lean proteins, along with the Glycaemic Index, it seems that we were only half right on both counts.

The role of carbohydrates

At any given moment the amount of carbohydrates in the adult body is about 300 grams or less. Some of this is in the blood, but most is stored in the liver and muscles as glycogen.

Carbohydrates have many functions; chief among them is to provide (1) energy to carry on the work of the body and (2) heat to maintain the body's temperature. Glucose, which is formed when carbohydrates are broken down, is the only form of energy used by the central nervous system, even though other tissues also use fats for energy.

Other Things Carbohydrates Do

1. Carbohydrates spare proteins. This means that with carbohydrates on hand the body need not burn protein from your diet or your body tissue (this means muscle!) to meet energy needs.
2. Carbohydrates aid in the manufacture of non-essential amino acids (refer to Chapter 8 on protein).
3. Carbohydrates are required for the complete oxidation of fats. When too little carbohydrates are available, some fatty acids known as ketones accumulate. A high accumulation of ketones is called ketosis, which interferes with the acid/base balance and causes the blood to become more acidic. Eventually, the condition known as ketoacidosis occurs, which can cause brain damage and eventually death. Dehydration is also a common consequence of ketosis because the body loses water-excreting ketones in the urine.
4. All carbohydrates except fibre have 4 calories per gram. fibre is not utilized for energy and therefore does not have a caloric value.

Is your glycaemic response making you fat?

Equal amounts of carbohydrates from different foods (such as sugar, pastas, legumes, and breads) can produce different increases in blood sugar (technically, blood glucose) in a given time. The immediate effect of carbohydrates on blood sugar is ranked on the Glycaemic Index (GI). As blood glucose levels rise, so does insulin, a hormone that helps shuttle blood glucose out of the blood and into the tissue cells to be used for energy. Insulin promotes fat storage—one reason that eating foods high on the Glycaemic Index tends to make you fat. Not only that, after your blood sugar rapidly rises, it will fall again sharply. The fall makes you feel hungry again, which can lead to overeating.

High insulin levels are associated with obesity.

Choosing carbohydrates wisely

Carbohydrates are an essential part of a healthy eating plan. The amount and type of carbohydrates you consume (using the Glycaemic Index as a guide for making healthy choices) will affect your fat-loss efforts.

The fact is, the modern diet is too rich in high-GI carbohydrates (those foods with a GI rating of 70 or higher). Common high-GI foods are cookies, crackers, bakery items, sweets, snack items, and simple sugars—some claiming to be low-fat or healthy! This is one of the major reasons that people are getting fatter and fatter, with Type 2 diabetes now showing up even in children, who will in turn become the next generation of obese adults.

Now is the time for high-profile nutritional education if we are to prevent a future health catastrophe.

It's never too late

It's never too late to change unhealthy eating habits. For example, middle-aged people accustomed to diets of high-GI foods can switch to low-GI foods (those foods with a GI rating below 55) and be far less likely to develop diabetes and heart disease. Examples of low-GI foods are fruits (apples, cherries, and pears), dairy products, stoneground or whole-grain products (oatmeal, brown rice, bulgur, and some cereals and breads), beans, and lentils.

Low-GI diets can also help control established diabetes by keeping blood glucose levels down. Low-GI diets also can help you lose weight, may lower blood lipids, improve the body's sensitivity to insulin, reduce the Glycaemic Index rating of the overall meal, and improve appetite control.

Additionally, low-GI carbohydrates satisfy your appetite without "over-satisfying" your caloric requirement. This idea is discussed in detail in *The New Glucose Revolution*, a widely acclaimed book on the detrimental effects of high-GI foods.

In the 3-Apple-a-Day GI Diet Substitution List (see page 157), you'll find that most carbohydrate foods are given a glycaemic rating. Following are the categories of low-, intermediate-, and high-GI rating of foods:

Low-GI rating	below 55
Intermediate-GI rating	between 55 and 70
High-GI rating	more than 70

Protein (meats, fish, and poultry) and fat (oils, nuts, and seeds) have little to no effect on glycaemic response and play a vital role in keeping the glycaemic response to a high-GI food to a minimum. In other words, you won't get hungry an hour later.

The vicious circle of high-GI foods

You might have heard that high-GI foods are used to replenish energy stores in endurance athletes. That is true. But for everyone else, high-GI foods are best minimized, since their primary contribution to the diet is empty calories.

In her book *Potatoes not Prozac*, Kathleen DesMaisons, PhD, writes about people who are unusually drawn to high-GI foods. She says that sugar sensitivity can cause people to consume large quantities of sweets, breads, pasta, or alcohol. These items can trigger feelings of exhaustion and low self-esteem, yet the spike and fall in blood sugar levels causes sugar-sensitive people to crave high-GI foods even more.

This seemingly endless cycle can continue for years, leaving sufferers overweight, fatigued, depressed, and sometimes alcoholic.

The 3-Apple-a-Day GI Diet is right on track

The primary carbohydrates in the 3-Apple-a-Day GI Diet are from low-GI and high-fibre sources. However, you will also find some intermediate- and high-GI sources included in some of the recipes. According to *The New Glucose Revolution*, mixing a high-GI food with a low-GI food yields an intermediate-GI meal.

Carbohydrate recommendations

The DRI, for both children and adults, is at least 130 grams of carbohydrates per day, based on the minimum needed to produce enough glucose for the brain to function.

The recommendation in the 3-Apple-a-Day GI Diet is that 40 per cent of total calories (which is 1 gram per pound of body weight) come from carbohydrates. This amount of carbohydrates is equal to the protein recommendation to establish your blood sugar levels and provide lasting energy throughout the day. Carbohydrate intake in the plan ranges from 128 to 187 grams per day (see Nutrient Chart for Fat Loss on page 62).

> **TIP:** When you eat carbohydrates that are not listed in the plan, choose those that have 2 to 4 grams of fibre per 100 calories. Whole grains, fruit, and vegetables are good sources of fibre.

Fibre—it does more than keep you regular

Dietary fibre is an edible, nondigestible component of carbohydrates naturally found in plant food. Also called "roughage" or "bulk", it has been recommended for years to maintain bowel regularity. Scientists and clinicians have also found that dietary fibre may reduce the risks of certain gastrointestinal diseases, diabetes, obesity, cardiovascular diseases, and colon or rectal cancers.

Two types of fibre

There are two general types of fibre, soluble and insoluble. Soluble fibre may help reduce the risk of heart disease. Insoluble fibre is essential for healthy digestion and may reduce the risk of gastrointestinal diseases.

Unlike most fruits, apples have high amounts of both soluble and insoluble fibre. So by eating apples you're getting not only a heart-healthy benefit but a gut-healthy one also!

Modern diets are lacking in fibre owing to the glut of highly processed, conveniently available foods. The typical diets that I have analyzed from seven-day food records averaged 10 to 13 grams of fibre per day. That is only one-third of both the DRI and American Cancer Society recommendations! Adding three apples per day will give you half of your fibre recommendation. Just add to that two or three servings of vegetables and your fibre requirement is met for the day.

Fibre recommendations

The DRIs for fibre range from 21 to 38 grams for adults, depending on age and gender. fibre in the 3-Apple-a-Day GI Diet ranges from 22 to 69 grams, depending on your calorie level (see Nutrient Chart for Fat Loss on page 62). This amount of fibre will keep your digestive tract healthy and accelerate your fat-loss efforts.

> **TIP:** Adding too much fibre too fast can cause bloating, wind, and cramps. If your diet has been low in fibre, gradually add fibre over several weeks to avoid discomfort.

CHAPTER 8

Protein—The Body's Building Blocks

The great protein debate

Nutrition experts have long sought the ideal combination of proteins, carbohydrates, and fats in respect to weight loss. Now with the return of the high-protein diets, protein consumption is being strenuously debated, alongside the conventional concerns about saturated fats (see Chapter 9 on fats) and cholesterol.

Do moderately high protein diets that are low in saturated fats and cholesterol (like the 3-Apple-a-Day GI Diet) raise the same concerns?

Study confirms the 3-Apple-a-Day GI Diet basics

A 10-week study led by Donald K. Layman, nutrition professor at the University of Illinois, found that women who ate 1,700 calories, with protein consumption based on body weight (0.73 gram of protein per pound of body weight), lost body fat, maintained muscle, and saw an improvement in total blood cholesterol. This group also reported being less hungry between meals, and they experienced stable blood glucose levels and reduced insulin response following meals.

By comparison, participants in the study's control group, who consumed half as much protein (0.36 gram per pound of body weight), lost significantly less body fat and were unable to maintain muscle mass.

Dr. David Katz, MD, author of *The Way to Eat*, confirms that eating enough protein maximizes calorie burning throughout the day. Research suggests that women who add 2 ounces of protein to each meal burn an extra 200 calories per day.

These studies confirm what I have found with various programs using the 3-Apple-a-Day GI Diet: My clients who consume 40 per cent of their calories from lean protein report they are *less hungry between meals and have more control over their appetites*. These clients also maintained muscle mass and lost more body fat than did those who didn't eat enough protein.

The function of protein in the body

The body uses proteins for building the structure of all cells, for the regulation of many body processes, and as a potential source of energy.

The protein structure of each type of tissue in the body is unique. Each body protein is constructed to perform specific functions and cannot be replaced by other proteins. Adequate protein levels in the diet are necessary for building new muscle tissue. Additionally, consuming protein at each meal provides a sense of satiety (feeling satisfied).

Proteins consist of chains of amino acids. Your body can make some of these amino acids (called non-essential amino acids), but other amino acids must be obtained from your diet (called essential amino acids). Essential and non-essential amino acids are each needed to build proteins that carry out the important functions of your body, such as creating new muscle, repairing tissue, manufacturing hormones, and regulating fluid balance.

How protein affects blood sugar levels

When protein foods are eaten, there is very little rise in blood sugar levels, which means there is very little rise in insulin levels. This is a good thing. The lower your insulin levels, *the less chance there is your body will want to store fat*.

Complete and incomplete proteins

Protein sources that contain all of the essential amino acids are called "complete proteins". Complete proteins are eggs, milk, cheese, meat, poultry, and fish.

Protein sources that lack one or more essential amino acids are called "incomplete proteins". Incomplete proteins are plant foods such as cereals and grains, beans, legumes, nuts, and vegetables. Incomplete proteins can be mixed and combined to make a "complete" protein. For example, the main source of protein for vegetarians comes from plants, so using a combination of incomplete proteins (such as beans and rice) fills the requirement. For vegetarians, it's difficult to achieve a perfect balance of carbohydrates to protein, mainly because the protein sources also contribute a high amount of carbohydrates. However, egg whites and fish are excellent non-carbohydrate sources of lean proteins.

Protein recommendations

The DRI for protein is that it make up 10 to 35 per cent of your total caloric intake. The 3-Apple-a-Day GI Diet recommends 40 per cent calories from protein, or 1 gram per pound body weight (see Nutrient Chart for Fat Loss on page 62). We have found that this amount of protein keeps your appetite under control and allows you to maintain valuable muscle tissue as you shed body fat.

> **TIP:** Include a small amount of a complete protein each time you eat.

CHAPTER 9

Fats—Healthy versus Unhealthy

Good for you or not?

Fat is associated with overweight. Billions of dollars are spent annually by people trying to lose excess layers of body fat. Yet controversy remains about the role dietary fats play in causing disease. Many believe lowering your fat intake will improve health. Others believe replacing "bad" fats with "good" fats will improve health.

Unfortunately, if you are overfat, it is likely that the amount of fat you burn is small, relative to the amount of fat you store. The more fat you eat—whether it is good or bad fat—the more fat you'll store. Luckily, this situation can be changed through diet and exercise, which is the goal of the 3-Apple-a-Day GI Diet.

Saturated fat versus unsaturated fat

For my Master's degree thesis, I compared the effects of saturated fats versus unsaturated fats on cholesterol and triglyceride levels in guinea pigs.

I created four diets for my pigs, two for each type of fat—

saturated and unsaturated. One diet was based on more of each fat (29 per cent of total calories) and one on less (19 per cent of total calories).

The guinea pigs eating the diet with more of either fat, saturated or unsaturated, had significantly higher visual internal body fat, especially around the organs (heart, liver, kidneys) than did the guinea pigs eating less fat, whether saturated or unsaturated.

But both groups that consumed either amount of saturated fats ended up with higher cholesterol compared with those who ate unsaturated fats. The triglyceride levels were not significantly different.

Although humans are not guinea pigs, we do metabolize fats similarly. What can we learn from my guinea pigs? That a high-fat diet makes you fat, even if the fat you eat is mainly "good" fat. Good fat in large amounts may leave your cholesterol low, but it won't make you thin.

Your body's fat requirements

Only a small amount of fat is needed for normal body function, and a lower-fat diet will aid in maximizing body-fat loss. According to Dr. Jequier, writing in the *European Journal of Clinical Nutrition*, to encourage normal body functions, fat intake should not be below *10 per cent of the total energy intake*.

How fat functions

Fat is a constituent of the body with its own functions, and researchers are beginning to think of it as more like an organ rather than just passive "insulation".

1. Dietary fats provide 9 calories per gram. (A tablespoon of oil is about 14 grams and 120 calories.) The body's deposits of fat

are a built-in reserve for energy, and we have an unlimited capacity for storing excess fat.

2. Fat (like carbs) is protein sparing because its availability reduces the need to burn protein for energy.
3. By providing insulation, fats help maintain a constant body temperature.
4. Fat provides cushion for the organs.
5. Fat facilitates the absorption of the fat-soluble vitamins A, D, E, and K.

Three classifications of fat

Fat may be saturated, polyunsaturated, or monounsaturated. Saturated fats have been associated with increased risk of heart disease. They mostly come from animal sources such as fatty meats and full-fat dairy products. Polyunsaturated and monounsaturated fats, which usually come from plant sources, have been associated with the reversal of heart disease.

But some plant oils are partially hydrogenated by manufacturers (an example is margarine) to form trans-fatty acids. Trans-fatty acids increase the risk of heart disease by boosting levels of LDLs (see the discussion of cholesterol in Chapter 10). Trans-fatty acids are not essential fats and provide no health benefits. The 3-Apple-a-Day GI Diet steers clear of these.

Why essential fats are . . . essential

Essential fats must be present in the diet because the body cannot make them. Two essential fatty acids are linoleic acid and linolenic acid.

Linoleic acid (omega-6 fatty acids), found in cottonseed oil, safflower oil, and sunflower oil, is required for normal growth, healthy skin, transport and metabolism of cholesterol, and other bodily functions. The omega-6s are all used heavily in processed foods such as crackers, cookies, crisps, and pastries. Although vital to cellular health, too many omega-6 fatty acids can negate the benefits of omega-3s.

Linolenic acid (omega-3 fatty acids) is found in salmon, tuna, sardines, ground flaxseeds, and flaxseed oils. According to Artemis Simopoulos, MD, director of the Center for Genetics, Nutrition, and Health, omega-3s have been found to counter a variety of illnesses and diseases. It is believed that the problem with our modern diet is that it contains far more omega-6 fatty acids than omega-3s, causing an imbalance, which makes us more vulnerable to many diseases. The 3-Apple-a-Day GI Diet is designed to help you achieve a good balance of these fatty acids.

Fat recommendations

The DRI for fat is 20 to 35 per cent of total calories. The 3-Apple-a-Day GI Diet includes 20 per cent of daily calories from fat (see Nutrient Chart for Fat Loss on page 62). This amount of fat meets your essential fat requirements, but doesn't provide unnecessary additional calories that would hinder your fat-loss efforts.

The DRI for essential fats per day are as follows: omega-6s, 12 grams for women and 17 grams for men; omega-3s, 1.1 grams for women and 1.6 grams for men.

> **TIP:** Fats are high in calories, very concentrated, and we need very little. Try to consume fats in their original form (for example, flaxseeds instead of flaxseed oil). To get the omega-3s you need, eat 3 ounces of salmon three times per week or add ground flaxseeds to cereal or protein shakes. When eating foods with labels, look for less than 2 grams of fat per 100 calories per serving.

CHAPTER 10

Cholesterol and Triglycerides

What is cholesterol?

Cholesterol is a waxy substance that is often confused with fat. Although cholesterol can be found in all high-fat foods, its main source is animals.

Cholesterol is a necessary and important substance in the body. It is a major structural component of all cells and is especially abundant in the nerve and brain cells. It becomes a problem only when it accumulates in the blood. Your total cholesterol level is made up of two measures: LDLs (low-density lipoproteins) and HDLs (high-density lipoproteins).

LDLs deliver cholesterol to the cells. They have been termed "bad" cholesterol because research shows that at high levels in your blood, they are associated with an increased rate of heart disease.

On the contrary, HDLs pick up cholesterol from arterial plaque, reducing accumulation. HDLs are termed "good" cholesterol because they appear to have a protective influence against heart disease.

Triglycerides, the technical name for fats and oils, are found in our food and our bodies. Triglycerides have many functions, such as transporting fat-soluble vitamins and providing an energy source (see the discussion of triglycerides that follows). But high levels of triglycerides *in the blood* are associated with diabetes and increased risk of heart disease. Following are the normal ranges for blood cholesterol and triglyceride levels:

Total cholesterol	< 200 mg/dl (milligrams per decilitre)
LDL	< 100 mg/dl
HDL	> 40 mg/dl
Triglycerides	< 150 mg/dl

What affects cholesterol and triglycerides?

Research has shown that eating high-cholesterol foods does not increase blood cholesterol levels in most people. In fact, less than 1 per cent of heart disease patients are actually affected by dietary cholesterol. But they *are* affected by saturated fats, which many high-cholesterol foods are loaded with. Take a close look at food labels and don't be reassured if that label says "no cholesterol". The item could still be loaded with either saturated fat or trans-fatty acids.

Research has shown that, as part of your total cholesterol, the LDL level is most influenced by your intake of saturated fats and trans-fatty acids, which cause a significant increase in cholesterol levels. Common food sources of these fats are full-fat animal products, cookies, crackers, bakery goods, snack items, and other convenience-type foods.

The goal of your diet should be to lower the LDLs and increase the HDLs. This can be done easily by exercising and losing excess body fat. Some research indicates that HDLs are also increased by consuming small amounts of alcohol. But before you run out and buy a cary-out, consider that other studies suggest that women may not experience the benefit.

Alcohol can also increase blood levels of triglycerides, as can high-GI carbohydrates such as sugar, corn syrup, and other simple sugars. Consuming such things is not very helpful if your goal is permanent fat loss.

Apples linked to heart health

A Finnish study of 5,133 men and women ages 30 to 69 concluded that a high consumption of flavonoids (a substance found in fruits) from apples was directly associated with the lowest risk for coronary mortality.

Another study from the University of California at Davis confirmed that important phytochemicals (from plants) in both apples and apple juice prevented oxidation (stickiness) of LDL cholesterol in the arteries. This stickiness causes buildup (plaque), which is harmful and can lead to heart attacks and/or strokes.

So eat apples for fat loss and better health—your heart will thank you for it!

CHAPTER 11

Energy, Water, and Alcohol

What are your body's energy requirements?

The total energy requirement of the body includes the basal metabolism (rate of expenditure of energy by the body at rest), the amount of voluntary activity, the influence of food, the environmental temperature, and the special needs for tissue building. I will refer to energy requirements as calories or caloric needs.

How many calories do you really need?

The amount of calories you need varies and is influenced by many things specific to you, such as your body size, gender, age, lean and body fat composition, body temperature, thyroid function, and growth needs. So you can see why one diet does not fit all—even though some of the books would have you think so!

There are several equations you can use to estimate caloric needs, depending on your goals. One, the Harris Benedict equation, uses height, weight, and age to determine basal energy expenditure and is mainly used in clinical practice. Another estimation equation, the one used in this plan, is based on current body weight multiplied by 10 (refer to the following Nutrient Chart for Fat Loss, below.

Example: 150 pounds × 10 = 1,500 calories

Energy requirements from equations are only estimations and may need to be adjusted, higher or lower, depending on your goals. As you become more active and develop your muscle tissue, you may require more calories. Also, once you have reached your fat-loss goal, you'll need to increase your calories to maintain it. This is because during the fat-loss process you are in a state of catabolism (breaking down fat); once you get to your

The 3-Apple-a-Day GI Diet
Nutrient Chart for Fat Loss

Weight (pounds)	Calories	Protein (grams)	Carbohydrate (grams)	Fat (grams)	Fibre (grams)	Water (10-ounce glasses)
110	1,200	110	110	35	25–35	7
120	1,200	120	120	27	25–35	8
130	1,300	130	130	29	25–35	8
140	1,400	140	140	31	25–35	9
150	1,500	150	150	33	25–35	9
160	1,600	160	160	35	25–35	10
170	1,700	170	170	37	25–35	10
180	1,800	180	180	40	25–35	11
190	1,900	190	190	42	25–35	11
200	2,000	200	200	44	25–35	12
220	2,200	220	220	48	25–35	13
240	2,400	240	240	53	25–35	14
260	2,600	260	260	58	25–35	15
280	2,800	280	280	62	25–35	16
300	3,000	300	300	67	25–35	17

weight-loss goal, you may have to increase calories to prevent further weight loss.

How low can your calories go?

Many people believe that to lose weight, you need to lower your intake of calories. This is only partially true. If you keep your calories at your basal energy needs (the minimal amount of calories your body needs to maintain normal function), increased activity and exercise can create the deficit for fat loss.

On the other hand, if your calories are too low to start with, meaning below your basal energy requirements, you will have difficulty making progress. Your body will adopt a survival mode, and *conserve and protect its fat stores!* The key is to feed your muscle and not feed your fat. The foods in the 3-Apple-a-Day GI Diet are designed to do this.

Eat when you're hungry

Pay attention to your hunger cues. Eat when you are truly hungry. True hunger is when your stomach is "growling" or "rumbling". Many times we are so busy that we don't pay attention to our body's cues.

Many people often skip breakfast because they don't feel hungry in the morning, but *eating breakfast can boost your metabolism and set your blood sugar levels for the day*. Once you establish a routine of eating breakfast every day, it will be difficult to skip this meal.

Caffeine or stimulants can also interfere with hunger cues. If you do consume caffeine, do so in moderation—one to two cups of coffee or other caffeinated beverages per day.

When you follow the 3-Apple-a-Day GI Diet, its three meals, two snacks, and three apples per day will provide your body with highly nutritious foods that will prevent your feeling hungry for long. Make sure you're consuming adequate calories so you don't become over-hungry.

> **TIP:** Start by consuming 10 calories per pound of body weight. If you are too full or feel like you are "stuffing" yourself, lower your total calories by 100 calories per day. If you feel hungry often, increase your total calories by 100 calories per day.

Water—you can't live without it!

Water is one of the most important nutrients in your life. You can survive for only a few days without it, although you can live weeks without food. Remember: Inadequate fluid intake will slow your body's ability to maximize body fat loss.

What water does for your body

In your blood, water helps transport glucose, oxygen, and fats to working muscles and carries away metabolic by-products, such as carbon dioxide and lactic acid. In the urine, water helps eliminate metabolic waste products. The darker the urine, the more concentrated the wastes. (Your goal should be urine that is light or colourless.) Your body loses water when you sweat, which is one way your body avoids heat buildup. In the saliva and gastric secretions, water helps digestion. Water also lubricates the joints and cushions organs and tissues.

How much water should you drink?

The general recommendations are eight 10-ounce glasses of water per day. I recommend 0.6 ounce per pound of body weight of water or non-caloric, non-caffeinated beverages. Yes, the latter items count in your total water consumption, too (see Nutrient Chart for Fat Loss on page 62).

Example (for a female):
150 pounds × 0.6 ounce = 90 ounces of water per day

> **TIP:** Try to stick with non-caloric beverages for your fluid intake. Do not drink your calories, except for the protein shakes and smoothies that are listed in this plan.

Can alcohol fit into a fat-loss program?

Alcohol delivers 7 calories per gram. Alcohol also interferes with normal blood sugar levels and fat metabolism. Frequent drinking results in adverse effects on muscle growth. Alcohol decreases protein synthesis and affects type 2 muscle fibres (strength-type fibres) more than type 1 (endurance-type fibres). Excessive alcohol consumption or binge drinking can result in decreased levels of testosterone and increased levels of cortisol (a muscle-destroying hormone), which has a direct effect on muscle cells and can result in significant muscle wasting.

That said, remember what your goals are. *Do you want to run to reach them—or walk?*

Alcohol recommendation

For a fat-loss effect, pass on the alcoholic beverages until you've reached your desired body fat level. When you're there, an occasional drink will probably not affect your success.

> **TIP:** At parties or bars, if you feel awkward without a drink, ask for sparkling water with a slice of lime or a non-alcoholic beer. No one will know the difference.

Your body is similar to your car

Imagine your body is your dream car. The type of fuel you put in will determine how well your car (or body) will run. Will you choose supreme fuel or the cheap stuff? Naturally, you would want your dream car to stay in mint condition and last for years. So you would maintain it well, provide it with water for cooling, give it oil for lubrication, and always fill its tank with the best fuel. Your body is similar. Your muscles are the engine that requires the necessary fuel (carbohydrates and protein), water (lots), and oil (sparingly) for cooling, lubrication, and myriad other vital functions.

Do this maintenance religiously, and your body (and your car) will run like a dream for your lifetime!

CHAPTER 12

The Metabolic Cost of Food and Meal Frequency

Eating takes energy!

When food is eaten, energy is required to digest and utilize the nutrients from that food. This is called the *metabolic cost*, or *thermogenic effect*, of food. Your body has to expend energy to process the protein, carbohydrates, and fats you derive from eating; and the food you consume, in turn, helps you continue normal bodily functions.

When you have adequate intake of these nutrients, your body will run efficiently and will be unlikely to store body fat. On the other hand, if you have excess intake of protein, carbohydrates, or fats, *your body will store the excess as body fat*. To make matters even worse, your body will then hang on to the fat and proceed to burn the excess carbohydrates and protein.

TIP: If you seem extra-hungry on some days, fill up on some additional protein and water and wait 20 minutes. If this doesn't satisfy you, add more vegetables or fruit.

Eat more to lose!

Timing is of the essence when you are trying to lose body fat. Start the 3-Apple-a-Day GI Diet with breakfast and eat every two to three hours. The meals are low in fat, so your body will burn the calories quickly.

As your muscle tissue develops, your metabolism will also increase, and you may get very hungry between meals. Small, frequent meals are a key to keeping your blood sugar and insulin levels stable and constant to maintain your maximum energy level—and minimize the chance that excess calories in a meal will be stored as fat.

Don't skip meals!

Skipping meals or depriving your body of food for long periods of time (other than sleeping) will cause it to access alternative fuel sources to maintain normal body functions. This means your body will use its reserves: first glycogen (stored carbohydrates), then muscle tissue (protein), and only last, unfortunately, fat.

If this cycle continues, your body will become very good and efficient at storing fat. It's the feast and famine theory. Over time, you will needlessly lose (shrink) your muscle tissue (which decreases your metabolism) and *store more and more body fat*. There's that vicious circle again!

TIP: Plan and prepare your meals ahead of time. Always take food (especially apples) with you in case you may be delayed. Don't skip meals; you may end up eating something your fat cells would love to store!

Breakfast of champions

There's no doubt breakfast is important. A long-term study from the University of California at Los Angeles (UCLA) School of Public Health has been following a sample population of 5,000 adults since 1965—about two-thirds of whom have reported their eating and behavioural habits for a decade.

Young adults who said they ate breakfast every day were only half as likely to be obese eight years later. They were equally unlikely to develop insulin resistance syndrome, a metabolic imbalance that can lead to weight gain, Type 2 diabetes, and heart attack.

Along with this, David Ludwig from Children's Hospital in Boston speculates that a good breakfast keeps blood sugar under control and filling up in the morning helps manage hunger later in the day.

Not just *any* breakfast will do

When Ludwig fed 12 obese teenage boys breakfast and lunch under controlled conditions, he discovered that even the choice between instant and old-fashioned oatmeal made a big difference in overeating.

The more rapidly digested, high-carbohydrate meals—including instant oatmeal with sugar—pumped up insulin in the blood and suppressed other hormones, leading to hunger and more eating later in the day.

> **TIP:** If you aren't typically hungry first thing in the morning, try exercising and then eat your breakfast, if your schedule allows. Otherwise, start with a small amount, such as two or three egg whites and some apple slices and work up to the recommended calories you need to consume at breakfast, according to the plan.

So what's the bottom line?

Whole-grain or high-fibre carbohydrates (fruits or vegetables) combined with a good source of protein (eggs, low-fat dairy products, or lean meats) as laid out in the 3-Apple-a-Day GI Diet provide lasting energy. Count on it!

You've reached your goal. Now what?

Oftentimes, losing weight is not as difficult as keeping the weight off (been there, done that?). So it's critical for you to understand as you go through your fat-loss phase that if you want to keep the fat off, most of the changes you've made have to be continued forever.

Yes, forever. *This is the secret to permanent fat loss.*

Why do people gain back their weight?

There are several explanations for the perplexing problem of regaining lost weight. One of the most common is that people lose weight too fast and a significant part of that weight is muscle. That's why you may want to focus on losing only 1 to 2 pounds per week.

Remember, 1 pound of fat equals 3,500 calories that need to be burned. That is a lot of energy to exert for just 1 pound of fat. If you are losing weight faster than that, it's likely you're losing muscle tissue. And as I've said before, losing muscle tissue makes it more difficult for you to burn off fat.

Another reason some people gain weight back is that they stop exercising once they attain their goal. You must realize that you can't just stop exercising and/or eating well and expect your body to maintain the same size and weight.

Finding the balance, as well as how much you can "get away with" (and not gain the weight back) can be tricky.

Tips from clients who have been successful in maintaining their weight loss

- Plan a splurge day (maybe a holiday) or one splurge meal (maybe once a week) during which you allow yourself to indulge in anything you want.
- Continue keeping your food journal no matter how off track you are—you will find a "U-turn" in the process.
- Keep exercising but scale back the workout some and take one day a week to rest.
- Introduce more variation into your meal plans while playing by the rules.
- Always keep your water intake on track.

Life goes on

So what if you lost your focus today? Get back on track with the next meal! Sometimes you have to live a little. You will always have opportunities such as birthdays, dinner parties, and holidays to eat foods other than what is listed in the plan.

The key is to keep in mind what you are striving for. Prepare ahead of time for entertaining, parties, and other food-related engagements so that you can continue to progress mentally and physically. When company comes to visit and stay with you, serve them what you would eat. If you are going to a party, eat before you go or eat lighter throughout the day, prior to the party, so you can try small amounts of the food being served. You can't stop living just because you want to shape up. It's how you prepare for tempting times that will keep you on track.

A lifetime commitment

View the 3-Apple-a-Day GI Diet as a journey or challenging adventure that will get easier as time passes, if you stay focused. I believe holidays (the official ones listed on the calendar—not ones you make up on your own!) are the time to splurge, and the rest of the time you should stay focused on keeping your body strong and healthy.

As a side benefit, those special events will be even more enjoyable, thanks to the self-confidence and pride that your new strong, healthy, good-looking body will bring to your life.

CHAPTER 13

Dining Out, Portion Control, Convenience, and Supplements

Let someone else do the cooking

Dining out can be an enjoyable experience, and there's no reason to hibernate when you are on a fat-loss program—especially when restaurants can easily fit into your meal plan.

All you have to do is follow the tips below and be firm when you order. Most restaurants are quite used to people on special diets and are happy to accommodate your needs. Remember, you are the one picking up the bill—and leaving the tip!

Tips for Dining Out

- Always order salad dressing on the side. Ask for low-calorie or fat-free dressing.
- With pasta, rice, or baked potato, ask for sauce, butter, sour cream, or other high-fat toppings on the side.
- When ordering meat, choose grilled chicken breast or fish rather than breaded or fried.

- Avoid deep-fried or fried foods. Not only are they loaded with fat and low in nutrients but they also usually contain trans-fatty acids or "bad" fats.
- Ask for stir-fry without oil.
- Instead of the regular side dishes, ask for a double order of steamed vegetables.
- At a Mexican restaurant, request whole beans instead of refried. Ask for cheese, sour cream, and guacamole on the side. Order chicken fajitas instead of beef and ask for corn tortillas instead of flour tortillas.
- At fast-food places, order a grilled chicken breast sandwich with sauce on the side or salads without the cheese and without regular salad dressing.
- Order pizza without cheese or cut the amount of cheese in half. Ask for vegetable toppings or lean Canadian bacon. Order extra-thin crust.

Super-size portions: more than you bargained for?

Our society wholeheartedly embraces the notion that bigger is better. You can "super-size" almost any fast-food item inexpensively—it's called "value marketing". It seems to make economical sense, too, as you get more food for very little extra cost. The real expense may come later if you have to deal with medical bills from overfat-related diseases. Unfortunately, you can't super-size your health care benefits these days.

A study conducted by health organizations nationwide, including the American Institute for Cancer Research, attempted to quantify how much damage value marketing does. Here are some of their findings:

- At McDonald's, researchers paid 8 cents *less* to buy the large value meal (Quarter Pounder with cheese, large fries, and large Coke at 1,380 calories) than a Quarter Pounder, small

fries, and small Coke (890 calories). In other words, for 8 cents *less* they purchased 490 more calories.

- When study participants ordered a medium popcorn without butter (900 calories) at the cinema, they were "upsold" to a large popcorn (1,160 calories) for only 60 cents more—it cost 23 per cent more for 260 more calories.
- At 7-Eleven, researchers asking for a "Gulp" of Coke (150 calories) left the store with a "Double Gulp" (600 calories) for only 37 cents more—a 42 per cent increase in price for *400 per cent more calories*.
- At another fast-food restaurant, a study participant asked for a cheeseburger and was upsold to a meal package—cheeseburger, fries, and Coke—for only $1.40 more. Even "better", she could super-size that meal for only 58 cents more. Her lunch now contained 1,380 calories, or about 700 more calories than a woman her size requires at lunch.

Are you portion challenged?

Food and beverage portions have grown over the past few years in restaurants, shop items, and even at home. Many people do not have any clue as to what a normal portion size should be.

So when you begin this plan, take the time to measure your food accurately—it's very important to get a realistic picture of what you're actually consuming. Use weighing scales, measuring cups, and measuring spoons. You'll soon begin to identify portion sizes just by looking. In fact, most people get the hang of it within a few weeks—and so will you!

Here are some other visual techniques for gauging portions if you are dining out:

1 serving of vegetables or fruit = a closed fist
1 ounce of cheese = two extended fingers

1 cup of dry cereal = a cupped hand
1 serving (3 ounces) of meat = the size of the palm of your hand
1 teaspoon of butter = the tip of your thumb

> **TIP:** Measure your foods accurately when you start this plan. Your efforts will yield worthwhile results.

Weight loss is not always "convenient"

We are becoming a fast-food nation, and our society seems to want more and more convenience. We have the technology to provide it, too; but this same convenience is one of the major contributing factors in making us fatter.

Achieving *permanent fat loss* sometimes is not convenient. Although the apples in this plan do provide convenience, learning to cook and prepare meals ahead of time will add even more convenience, not to mention better taste—and you'll know what's in the food you're eating!

> **TIP:** Use your supermarket, not the drive-through window, as a source for wholesome foods.

Potato chips and couch potatoes

I wrote a letter to the President of the United States last year asking for a nationwide, federally funded, Get-in-Shape Contest. The purpose was to help combat the escalating obesity problem by motivating people to get off their couches, put on their gym shorts—and eat more fruits and vegetables.

Did you know that the majority of marketing money is spent on junk food (which makes us fatter) and the least amount is spent on marketing produce (fruits and vegetables)? Yet we scratch our heads and wonder why people are getting fatter—not to mention more sedentary. Hello?

More fat people are on the way, too. You'll see why if you ever watch TV programming for kids, which features one junk-food commercial after another (with no fruits and vegetable commercials at all!).

Although I did not get a reply from the President, anyone can write to their MP and make suggestions for national health improvements. If enough people speak up, someone will hear.

Do you need supplements to succeed?

Not on the 3-Apple-a-Day GI Diet. As a dietitian, I believe food is the best source of fuel for optimizing your fat loss. Food is what helps our body repair itself. However, with the lower daily caloric intakes (1,200 or 1,500), I do recommend a multivitamin and mineral supplement and additional calcium for most people, even if their diet is the best it can be.

A vitamin, mineral, and calcium supplement is not a replacement for a poor diet but an enhancement to a very good diet. In this plan, I suggest a shake that requires protein powder. This is primarily for convenience and not a necessity. You can substitute the protein shake for another snack or meal choice.

As for other sports-enhancement supplements, I do not recommend that you use them in your efforts to maximize fat loss. Many of the fat-loss products or thermogenics on the market are not regulated by the US Food and Drug Administration (FDA) and may be unsafe. I recommend apples as your fat-loss supplement to keep your hunger under control.

A moderate intake of caffeine (one to two cups of coffee per day, or 300 milligrams of caffeine) can enhance both performance and endurance. Caffeine releases free fatty acids, which can provide additional energy for your workout. On the other hand, too much caffeine can interfere with the body's absorption of calcium and other nutrients. Too much caffeine can also delay the hunger response (your cue to eat), which may cause you to overeat later in the day.

TIP: Eating equal amounts of protein and carbohydrate plus exercising will give you the greatest fat loss results.

Key Points for Part III

- Aim for each meal to include a fruit and/or vegetable, lean protein, and water.
- Consume 1 gram each of lean protein and low-GI carbohydrate per pound of body weight per day.
- Your fibre intake should be at least 25 to 35 grams per day. Three apples provide 15 grams alone.
- Eat 3 ounces of salmon, tuna, sardines, trout, or mackerel, three times per week, to get your essential fats.
- Start by consuming 10 calories per pound of your current weight as your total daily calorie intake.
- Drink at least eight 10-ounce glasses of water per day.
- Eat breakfast and four to five small meals every day to keep your metabolism and energy level optimum.
- Measure your food in the beginning to ensure accurate portions.
- Use apples as your fat-loss supplement, one before each major meal.

PART IV

EXERCISE: A KEY TO STAYING YOUNG

CHAPTER 14

Physical Activity versus Exercise for Permanent Fat Loss

So there's a difference?

Actually, yes. Recently, there have been several recommendations for the amount and types of exercise or physical activity needed to be healthy and/or to experience weight loss. Specialists have long advised 30 minutes of moderately intense physical activity every day for overall health. Recently, the new physical activity goal recommended by the US Institute of Medicine (author of the DRIs) is one hour per day, seven days per week. This recommendation is based on how much energy is expended from an individual of a healthy weight.

Physical activity includes walking the dog, house cleaning, stair climbing, playing catch with the kids, and other "moving" activities. Exercise is an exertion of mind and body for development and training. Exercise is being consciously active with a purpose. But all physical activity can increase your fat-loss efforts.

Exercise is work! When can I lighten up?

Let's clear the air on the whole exercise issue. It's not a temporary activity you do when you are on a "diet." To achieve *permanent fat loss*, you need to activate and build your lean muscle tissue—and maintain it throughout your life. There's just no getting around it!

My grandmother, 91 years young, lives alone and exercises at the gym three times per week and can out-walk any 50-year-old in town. Not only that, she's in better health, both mentally and physically, than many 50-year-olds! By the way, she eats at least one apple per day and includes fruits and vegetables with every meal.

Increasing your muscle tissue increases your metabolism, or metabolic rate (your ability to burn calories). The more you increase your muscle tissue, and therefore your metabolism, the more calories you'll burn—even while you are sleeping!

Your body was designed to be active. Today's environment has made it too easy to be sedentary—long commutes, lifts, computer-dominated jobs, remote controls, video games, the list goes on and on. According to the Centers for Disease Control and Prevention (CDC), nearly four out of ten adults report getting no exercise at all! Despite the legitimate worry over super-sized portions and junk food, some scientists argue that the obesity epidemic is mostly due to inactivity.

So let's get moving!

Two types of exercise

Basically, there are two major types of exercise your body needs for permanent fat-loss results: weight training and cardiovascular training. Stretching, functional training (moving in all ranges of motion with weights), and other types of training (martial arts, yoga, etc.) are also important additions for cross-training. All activity is good!

WEIGHT TRAINING

Weight training, or resistance exercise, is used to strengthen the muscles and maintain or increase muscle tissue. One of the biggest benefits of weight training is that you "wake-up" muscle cells that would not otherwise be activated with any other exercise. This creates more metabolically active tissue and increases your body's ability to burn calories. Weight training also strengthens the muscles around your bones, making you less prone to injury.

Many people (especially women) believe that weight lifting will give them big, bulky muscles. Although there are some who will develop obvious muscle faster, it's not likely that you will get big and bulky. The key is activating the muscle tissue and losing the fat layer on top of the muscle so you will have a leaner, sleeker body.

Research at the University of Alabama shows that just three strength-training sessions per week can help you burn 150 more calories every day—enough to shed 16 pounds of body fat a year.

Keeping your muscle tissue as you age is the key to staying active so you don't become disabled! After the age of 25, we can lose about 1 per cent of muscle mass per year (see the example in Chapter 3). According to Tufts University scientists, muscle loss is more universal than osteoporosis. As you lose muscle, you lose strength. When you lose strength, you lose the ability to be active and energetic. With weight training, you can increase your muscle mass at any age.

In other words, use it or lose it.

CARDIOVASCULAR TRAINING

Cardiovascular training strengthens the heart and improves the efficiency of the cardiovascular and respiratory systems. Certain cardiovascular exercises, termed "weight bearing" (bearing your own body weight)—brisk walking, running, dancing, stair climbing, and playing sports with your kids—can help keep you fit and promote bone mass. Best of all, if you are on a mission to lose weight, cardiovascular training is very effective in helping you lose that stubborn, unhealthy extra fat layer.

Train according to your fitness level

Weight training and cardiovascular training should both be gauged according to your fitness level. If you're a beginner, you'll need to condition your muscles, joints, and tendons gradually. If you've weight trained in the past but haven't been active for a while, you can ease into it over a few weeks. If you've been consistent with an exercise program, you may be ready to take it to the next level.

Always check with your GP before starting an exercise program, especially if you have had previous health risks.

Exercise recommendations

Beginner: train with weights three times per week starting with lighter weights and higher repetitions. Cardiovascular

TIP: If you are currently inactive, try using a pedometer (a device that measures every step you take) to determine your level of activity. You can find a pedometer at most department and sport shops (costs range from £10 to £30). Studies have shown that individuals who are at a healthy weight take at least 10,000 steps per day.

training should be performed four to five times per week for 20 minutes per day. As you become more fit, you'll need to increase your intensity (effort) and weights.

Intermediate: train with weights three to four times per week. You'll want a program that is progressive and has a variety of exercises, repetitions, and sets. Cardiovascular training should be performed five times per week for 30 to 40 minutes per day.

Advanced: train with weights four times per week with heavier weights and fewer repetitions. Perform cardiovascular training five to six days per week for 30 to 45 minutes per day.

The next chapter includes a beginner exercise program to get you started.

> **TIP:** Think of exercise as your prescription for survival. If you don't exercise, you'll shorten your active life. All activity and movement, from house cleaning to weight training, is cumulative and will improve your health.

The 3-Apple-a-Day GI Diet
Exercise Guidelines for Fat Loss

Level	Weight Training Sessions (per week)	Cardiovascular Training Sessions (per week/time)	Stretching Sessions (per week)
Beginner	3	4–5/20 minutes	5
Intermediate	4	5/30–40 minutes	5
Advanced	4	5–6/30–45 minutes	7

CHAPTER 15

A 12-Week Beginner's Exercise Program

Getting started

The exercise program I've created for you here assumes that you have had little regular exercise experience. This is just one idea for a simple three-day-a-week plan to get you started.

Begin each exercise session with a five-minute warmup and stretch. Warming up includes walking in place or using your favorite cardio equipment (treadmill, step machine, etc.); climbing stairs; or doing jumping jacks, twisting, and/or arm circles. Follow your warmup with light stretching.

Repetitions

"Repetitions" (or reps) refers to the number of times you actually move the weight through your full range of motion. If you lift your child from the ground to overhead 10 times in a row before resting, you have performed 10 repetitions of "child presses"! Your repetitions will increase as the weeks go by. Over time, you will also be increasing the amount of weight you use. If you can complete your sets and repetitions with good form, increase your weight on your next workout by about 5 per cent.

Sets

A "set" is a group of repetitions. The number of sets recommended is listed before the number of repetitions for that set (for example, 2 × 12, or two sets of 12 repetitions each). You would normally rest after each set. It is recommended that you rest for only 60 to 90 seconds (or more, if needed, when you are beginning).

Keeping an exercise journal

An exercise journal can be a great tool to record your progression as you become more fit. You can use it to keep track of the exercises you do each day and as a checklist to ensure that you are working your whole body. There are variations of exercises that work your muscles (strengthening exercises such as lunges and biceps curls) and your cardiovascular system (walking on the treadmill, stepping, etc.). The Weekly Exercise Tracking sheet on page 220 is a tool you can use to record your progress.

Work out at home or at a health club

The 12-Week Beginner's Exercise Program can be performed in a health club or at home. Many people like the convenience of working out at home. If you plan to work out at home, I suggest getting some inexpensive hand weights, ranging in weight from 3 to 12 pounds. You can also use 5-pound bags of sugar or flour, or fill empty one-gallon milk jugs with water (9 pounds) to use for weights. The key to any weight-training program is that you use resistance against the muscle for strengthening benefits. There are also many videos that can safely lead you through various exercises, such as sculpting, stretching, yoga, Pilates, and low-impact aerobics. Mix up your workout to keep things fresh!

Key Points for Part IV

- Physical activity and exercise are essential for permanent fat loss.
- Weight training will increase lean muscle tissue. Increasing muscle tissue will increase metabolism.
- Cardiovascular training will help you lose your existing excess fat layer.
- All physical activity will contribute to your fat-loss efforts and improve your health. Inactivity contributes to being overfat.

The 3-Apple-a-Day GI Diet
Twelve-Week Beginner's Exercise Program

Day	Exercise*	Weeks 1–2	Weeks 3–4	Weeks 5–6
Monday	Squats	1×8[†]	2×8	2×10
	Lunges	1×8	2×8	2×10
	Dumbbell chest press	1×8	2×8	2×10
	Triceps push-downs	1×8	2×8	2×10
	Ab[‡] crunches	1×20	2×20	2×25
	Cardiovascular[§]	15 minutes	20 minutes	25 minutes
	Stretching	5 minutes	5 minutes	5 minutes
		Weeks 7–8	**Weeks 9–10**	**Weeks 11–12**
	Squats	3×12	3×12	3×15
	Lunges	3×12	3×12	3×15
	Dumbbell chest press	3×12	3×12	3×15
	Triceps push-downs	3×12	3×12	3×15
	Ab crunches	3×25	3×30	3×30
	Cardiovascular	30 minutes	35 minutes	35 minutes
	Stretching	5 minutes	5 minutes	5 minutes
		Weeks 1–2	**Weeks 3–4**	**Weeks 5–6**
Tuesday	Cardiovascular	15 minutes	20 minutes	30 minutes
	Stretching	5 minutes	5 minutes	5 minutes
		Weeks 7–8	**Weeks 9–10**	**Weeks 11–12**
	Cardiovascular	30 minutes	40 minutes	40 minutes
	Stretching	5 minutes	5 minutes	5 minutes
		Weeks 1–2	**Weeks 3–4**	**Weeks 5–6**
Wednesday	Leg press	1×8	2×8	2×10
	Leg curls	1×8	2×8	2×10
	Lat pull-downs	1×8	2×8	2×10
	Dumbbell biceps curls	1×8	2×8	2×10
	Reverse crunch (abs)	1×20	2×20	2×25
	Cardiovascular	15 minutes	20 minutes	25 minutes
	Stretching	5 minutes	5 minutes	5 minutes
		Weeks 7–8	**Weeks 9–10**	**Weeks 11–12**
	Leg press	3×12	3×12	3×15
	Leg curls	3×12	3×12	3×15
	Lat pull-downs	3×12	3×12	3×15
	Dumbbell biceps curls	3×12	3×12	3×15

	Reverse crunch (abs)	3×25	3×30	3×30
	Cardiovascular	30 minutes	35 minutes	35 minutes
	Stretching	5 minutes	5 minutes	5 minutes
		Weeks 1–2	**Weeks 3–4**	**Weeks 5–6**
Thursday	Cardiovascular	15 minutes	20 minutes	30 minutes
	Stretching	5 minutes	5 minutes	5 minutes
		Weeks 7–8	**Weeks 9–10**	**Weeks 11–12**
	Cardiovascular	30 minutes	40 minutes	40 minutes
	Stretching	5 minutes	5 minutes	5 minutes
		Weeks 1–2	**Weeks 3–4**	**Weeks 5–6**
Friday	Squats	1×8	2×8	2×10
	Lunges	1×8	2×8	2×10
	Overhead press	1×8	2×8	2×10
	Push-ups	1×8	2×8	2×10
	Ab crunches	1×20	2×20	2×25
	Cardiovascular	15 minutes	20 minutes	25 minutes
	Stretching	5 minutes	5 minutes	5 minutes
		Weeks 7–8	**Weeks 9–10**	**Weeks 11–12**
	Squats	3×12	3×12	3×15
	Lunges	3×12	3×12	3×15
	Overhead press	3×12	3×12	3×15
	Push-ups	3×12	3×12	3×15
	Ab crunches	3×25	3×30	3×30
	Cardiovascular	30 minutes	35 minutes	35 minutes
	Stretching	5 minutes	5 minutes	5 minutes
		Weeks 1–2	**Weeks 3–4**	**Weeks 5–6**
Saturday	Cardiovascular	15 minutes	20 minutes	25 minutes
and Sunday	Stretching	5 minutes	5 minutes	5 minutes
		Weeks 7–8	**Weeks 9–10**	**Weeks 11–12**
	Cardiovascular	30 minutes	35 minutes	35 minutes
	Stretching	5 minutes	5 minutes	5 minutes

*Ask a trainer for a proper demonstration of these exercises or other exercise programs. You may get different recommendations from a trainer. That's OK, trainers have good reasons for their recommendations!

†Sets times repetitions: 1x8 = one set of eight repetitions.

‡Ab (abdominal) crunches.

§Walking, cycling, running, doing jumping jacks, jumping rope, climbing stairs, doing exercise videos, or using cardiovascular exercise machines.

PART V

SUCCESS STORIES

Nicole Szeghalmi, age 27

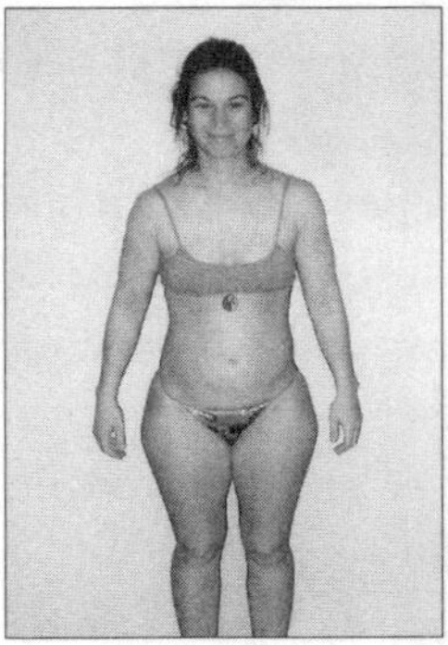

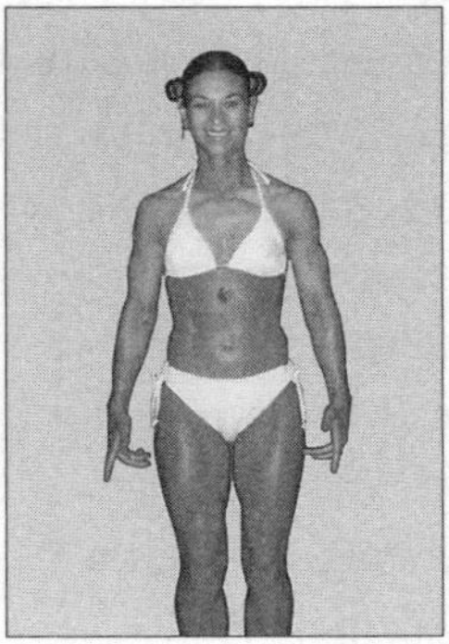

	Before	**After**	***Change***
Weight (pounds)	140	107	−33
Body fat (per cent)	26	11	−15
Waist (inches)	32	24	−8
Hips (inches)	40	33	−7
Thigh (inches)	24	19	−5

I owe the success of sticking with a sound nutrition plan (the 3-Apple-a-Day GI Diet) to apples. They were the foundation of my food program. There isn't any type of apples I haven't tried. As long as they're fresh, I'm happy.

The toughest time for me to stick to my healthy eating program was during the evening. I just love to snack at night. So I used apples to satisfy my snack cravings. The apples quieted the rumblings in my belly without weighing me down with a bunch of calories.

Every aspect of my life has improved. The 12-week "challenge" has had such a positive impact on the way I live my life that the list may cause me to run out of paper. Here are the top seven improvements I've seen:

1. *Knee pain:* I have had two surgeries and have been living daily with knee pain until now. I think the combination of losing weight and building strength gave my knee better support, relieving the pain.
2. *Ability to self-motivate:* I now believe that with hard work and dedication, I can accomplish any goals I set for myself.
3. *Skin complexion:* Because of my food program, my complexion has cleared up, and it looks healthy.
4. *Increased energy:* I have a lot of energy throughout the day now, whereas before I was taking naps.
5. *Increased strength:* I love how I can qualitatively track my progress with weights. In the beginning, I could barely lift 10-pound dumbbells while performing lunges, and now I can handle 30 pounds!
6. *Increased feeling of well-being:* Since I have been working out, my mood has improved, giving me a higher ability to cope with stresses, both good and bad. Therefore, I have a more positive outlook on life.
7. *Increased self-confidence:* My clothes seem to fit better now, and I don't feel like running and hiding when I have my bikini on.

So now I come to an end with this awesome experience. "Life-changing experience" would better describe it, and I have nothing but positive words and thoughts about it. I can't believe how fast the 12 weeks have passed. Although it was tough at times, I wouldn't trade it for anything. I look forward to new challenges.

Nicole won first place and $50,000 in the National Gold's Gym Challenge, 2003.

Stacey Lienemann, age 22

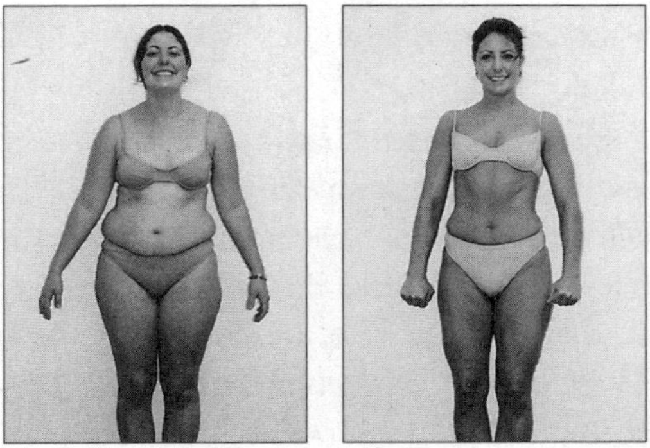

	Before	**After**	***Change***
Weight (pounds)	172	143	−29
Body fat (per cent)	33	21	−12
Waist (inches)	35.5	31.25	−4.25
Hips (inches)	44.25	38	−6.25
Thigh (inches)	26	23	−3

The Gold's Gym Challenge has changed my life dramatically. It's hard to imagine that a short 12 weeks ago I was an unhappy, unhealthy, and overweight 23-year-old mother of one, Jaden, my daughter who is sixteen months old.

I have always imagined myself as an active, happy mother with bounds of energy, strength, and creativity. Twelve weeks ago, I found myself at 172 pounds, tired, angry, and unhappy with my life. My family was suffering because of the way I was. My dream was to change my activities and eating habits to enable me to become healthier, both physically and mentally.

I knew that if I didn't do something to change my life soon I might never change it at all. Going through life unhappy and lazy is one of my biggest fears. That fear is what pushed me into the gym. I decided to join the Get-in-Shape Contest.

I put myself on a six-day-a-week workout plan that consisted of attending a variety of different classes. I also incorporated up to an hour of cardio a day.

I expected the beginning days to be gruelling. Lack of self-esteem, energy, and strength makes everything seem difficult. However, my drive and determination to become healthier and more physically fit motivated me tremendously. I didn't want to be the girl in the back of the class who gets winded after the warmup. So I stuck with it, and before long I began to gain strength and endurance. When I finished a class, I could feel my self-esteem grow and my bum shrink. The stronger I grew, the more I was able to push myself. The classes enabled me to have fun with my workout, and having a set time to be at the gym gave me the discipline I needed to continue my progress.

When it comes to dieting, discipline is my major problem. Eating has always been a challenge for me because I eat when I'm bored. When I'm not bored, I'm busy and I forget to eat altogether.

The 3-Apple-a-Day GI Diet made me realize what our bodies need to function. Realizing that food is fuel for your body helped me change my eating habits forever. Now instead of eating because I'm bored, I eat to fuel my muscles and produce energy. The more knowledge I gain about food and what it does for our bodies, the easier it is to pick healthy food choices.

In the past 12 weeks, I have become addicted to going to the gym first thing every day. My life has changed tremendously because of this contest. I love myself now, and that is the best prize I could ever receive. I can feel my dreams starting to come true. I am a fit, motivated, happy 23-year-old mother of one, and I am extremely proud of myself for accomplishing my goals.

Stacey won first place and $2,200 in Gold's Gym of Wenatchee local contest, 2003.

Jason Mathews, age 27

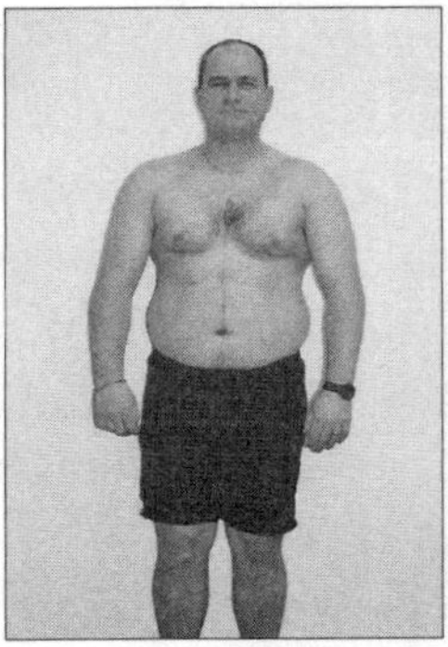

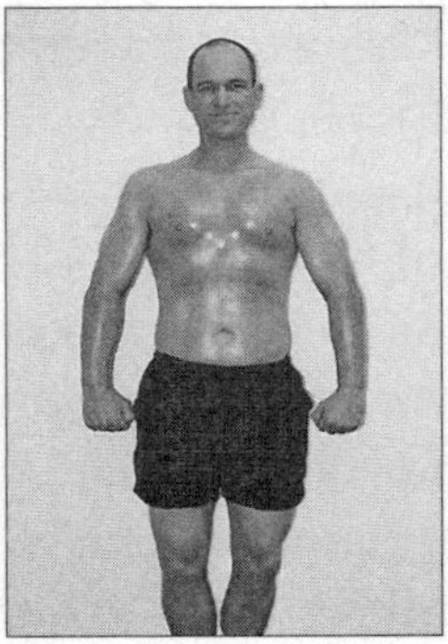

	Before	After	*Changes*
Weight (pounds)	258	199	−59
Body fat (per cent)	42	11	−31
Waist (inches)	45.75	36	−9.75
Hips (inches)	46.5	40.5	−6
Thigh (inches	29.5	24	−5.5

I had two big motivators to join the contest, my dad and my wife. About two years ago, my dad was diagnosed with diabetes and a large cancerous tumour on one of his kidneys. He had to make an immediate lifestyle change—eating healthier, exercising, and losing weight. He has been successful and is cancer free.

My wife was diagnosed with leukaemia over three years ago. At 25, this was a total shock to both of us. The treatment damaged her hip and required a hip replacement. Through her entire ordeal, we both gained a lot of weight.

I used to be involved in sports and activities and believed I was still in OK shape. Then I had a body composition test that revealed just how out of shape I had become. I was determined to get back into shape. My wife and I began our quest to become fit together.

What I really enjoyed was the immediate results from the diet and exercise program provided to us by Gold's Gym. I lost 12 pounds the first week. I always thought food had to have grease and fat to taste good, until we began cooking some of the recipes, especially the chilli, provided by Tammi Flynn. My wife and I both learned how to use fresh fruits and vegetables in our diet. We now plan and prepare foods to take with us to work.

During the contest, my wife and I learned a lot about willpower. If one of us thought about cheating, the other quickly steered that person back in the right direction.

The best thing now is to hear people ask my wife and me how much weight we have lost. And telling us that we look great!

Jason lost 85 pounds of fat and gained 26 pounds of muscle! He won first place and $2,200 in Gold's Gym of Wenatchee's local contest, 2003.

Vicki Robins, age 32

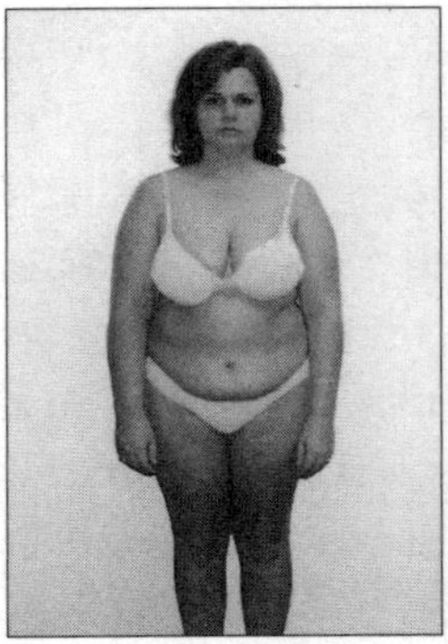

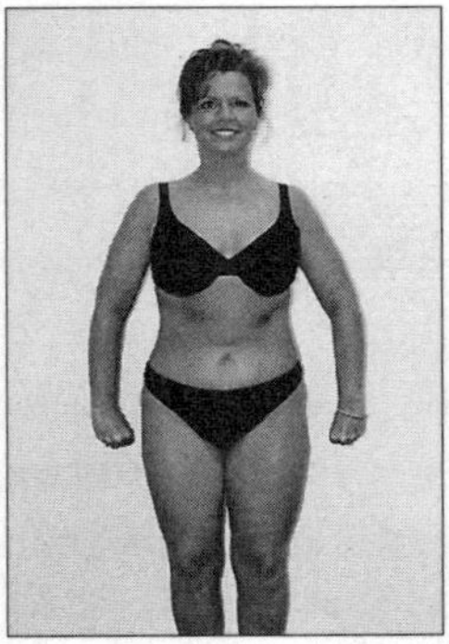

	Before	After	*Changes*
Weight (pounds)	158	134	−24
Body fat (per cent)	39	30.5	−8.5
Waist (inches)	40.25	32.5	−7.75
Hips (inches)	41.5	38	−3.5
Thigh (inches)	26	23.25	−2.75

"Mommy, if having babies in your tummy makes it big like yours, I don't want to have any," said my six-year-old daughter. I knew then that I needed to do something to change my eating habits. It is one thing to accept the image of a frumpy mom of three, but to hear these words is a big eye opener and very painful. I never knew my being overweight affected my children this way. I am a stay-at-home mom and give my children all of me, but I did not realize that in a sense that was too much. I want to be a positive role model in every way to my children, and the weight I was at was harming not only me but them as well.

When I looked at my "before" pictures, I was amazed and disgusted at how I had let myself go. The front pose is something I looked at every day and I had become used to it, but the back pose shocked me! This was the biggest motivator I needed. The times I felt like giving up, I just looked at my pictures, and that kept me going.

The words "discipline versus willpower" were constant in my thoughts. Also the pictures from past contestants gave me a boost when I needed one. To know that moms just like me had greatly improved their figures, I knew I too could do the same.

When I began eating healthier, everyone in my family benefited. I went from buying 21 apples per week to double that amount. My oldest daughter began reading labels and made sure I did not eat anything that was unacceptable to my new way of eating.

We, as a family, are also more active. All five of us are starting softball and loving the exercise together.

In 12 weeks, I attained all of my goals and then some. My daughter now realizes it is a choice to be frumpy and not a result of pregnancy. I find I am a better wife and mother for it and hope that my children will understand the importance of fitness. I can't wait to see what the next 12 weeks will bring. If I can do it, anyone can!

Vicki won first place and $2,200 in Gold's Gym of Wenatchee's local contest, 2003.

Tim Kiele, age 35

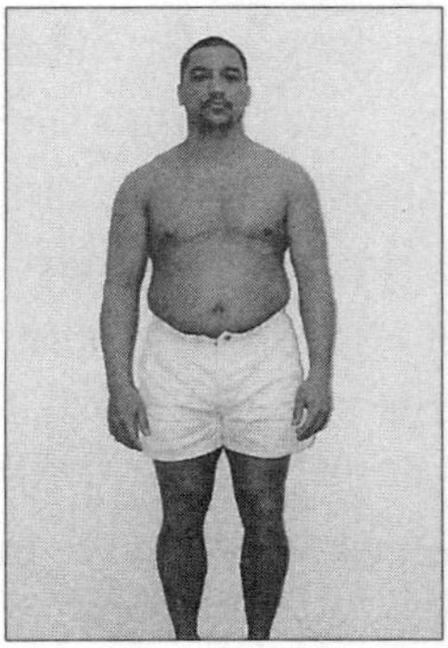

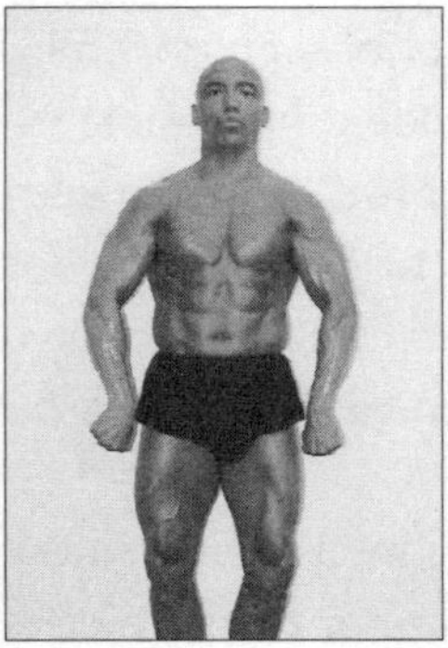

	Before	After	*Changes*
Weight (pounds)	178	155	−22
Body fat (per cent)	15	7	−8
Waist (inches)	37.25	31.5	−5.75
Hips (inches)	41	36	−5
Thigh (inches)	24.75	23	−1.75

There are several reasons that I chose to take the "challenge" at Gold's Gym. A neck injury, accompanied by bulging discs in my lower back, have hindered my life and the needs of my family.

Twelve years ago, when I met my wife, I played national flag football, basketball, softball, and golf. My dream was to become a daddy, and I was blessed with twin daughters. Never did I think I would have to utter the words "Sorry babies, Daddy's back hurts and he can't play right now." This had to stop. I owed it to my wife and children to change my life around.

During this contest, I have noticed dramatic changes in my body, which I attribute to the 3-Apple-a-Day GI Diet. Implementing apples alone was a step in the right direction. Eating apples caused me to eat less, and they are a great substitute between meals. I will continue to eat them on a daily basis!

I had a lot of support throughout the contest. Working graveyard has made it impossible to get a "good night's sleep". So one could imagine the challenge on some days—just making it to the gym, let alone getting in a good workout. The smiles and support of the staff created such positive energy that it gave me the boost I needed to push even harder toward the goals I had set for myself.

Those 12 weeks, through the contest, have given me back that "fire" I had prior to my injuries. Now that I have reached all my personal goals, I intend on setting future goals, which include helping my family live a healthier and happier lifestyle with me.

Tim won first place and $2,200 in Gold's Gym of Wenatchee's local contest and third place in the national Gold's Gym Challenge, 2003.

Maureen Ropp, age 48

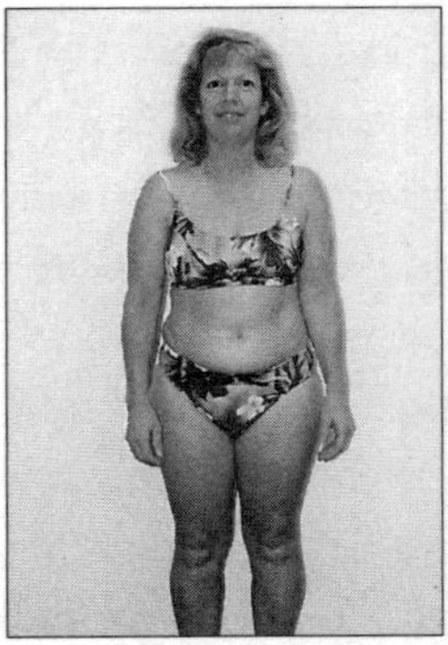

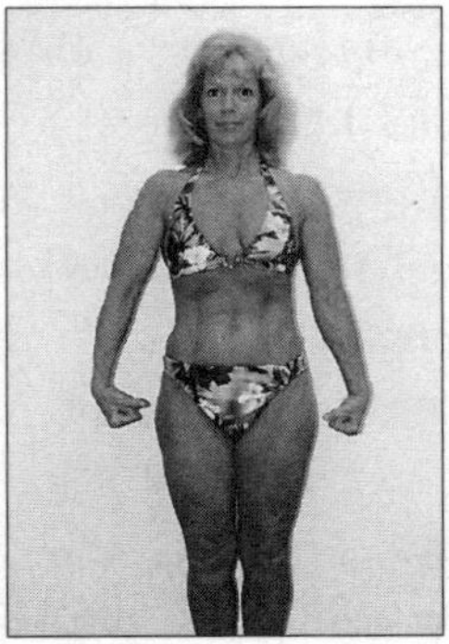

	Before	After	*Changes*
Weight (pounds)	143	120	−23
Body fat (per cent)	32	23	−9
Waist (inches)	32.75	29.25	−3.5
Hips (inches)	41	36	−5
Thigh (inches)	24.5	22	−2.5

I started this contest with my husband because we wanted to be healthier, and we could see ourselves gradually going in the wrong direction. We didn't want our physical health to limit what we could do—we wanted to choose our own lifestyles, our health, our own future and quality of life!

We found that *planning and preparation* is the key to success. We kept journals for our training, plus we used a program to track our calorie intake. We found we needed to measure and weigh everything until we learned proper portion sizes. We ate five to six meals per day and ate our three apples every day (my favourite is Fuji). We kept our fat intake to less than 20 per cent of our total calories and balanced our remaining calories between carbohydrates and protein (as in the 3-Apple-a-Day GI Diet). I have been very fortunate to have a very supportive husband who has helped me with training and food preparation. It's also great to have support from your family and friends.

We have set a personal goal of riding the 200-mile STP (Seattle to Portland) bike ride in July. I never imagined two years ago that I would be able to accomplish even a 20-mile ride. I was winded just climbing the stairs and my joints were starting to swell with soreness. Now I'm climbing hills with my bike!

If you learn how good you can feel and how much you can accomplish, regardless of age, then you definitely are a winner! I know I am!

Maureen won first place and $2,200 in Gold's Gym of Wenatchee's local contest, 2003.

Pete Faulkner, age 40

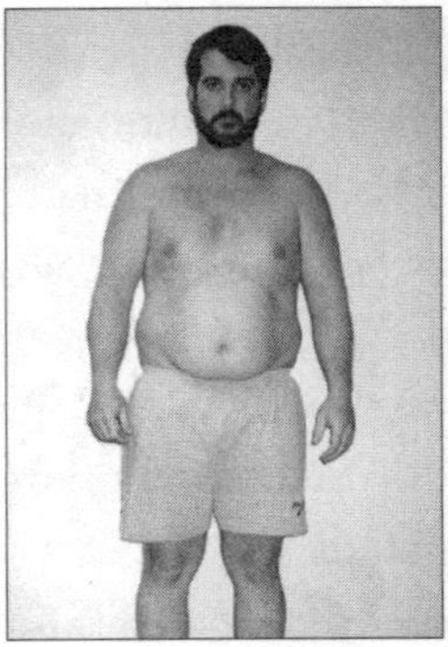

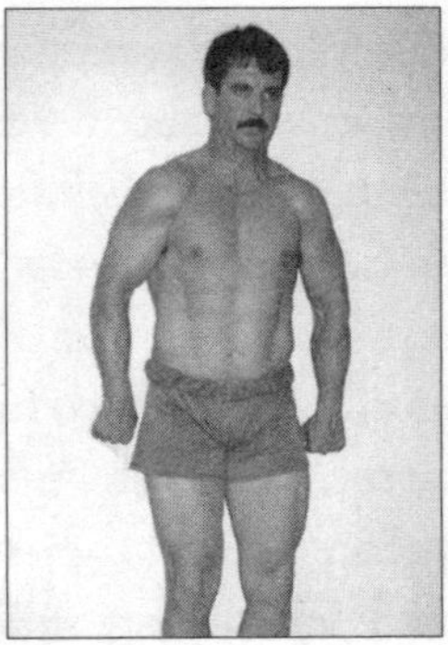

	Before	After	*Changes*
Weight (pounds)	215	173	−42
Body fat (per cent)	28	9	−19
Waist (inches)	45	34	−11
Hips (inches)	45.5	38	−7.5
Thigh (inches)	29	23.5	−5.5

I am a bricklayer by trade, as my father was and his father as well. I was raised among men, what you would call a "man's man". I've been married for 16 years to a beautiful wife who gave me two children and stuck with me through thick and thin. I felt my wife needed more of a husband and father than what I had become.

I was 50 pounds overweight. It hurt to get up in the morning. I could barely lay brick all day. After work all I could do was lay on the couch and watch TV. My children needed me to communicate and be active, but the energy just wasn't there. I would toss and turn all night. Some mornings I was more tired when I got up than when I had gone to bed. I was constantly ornery. I ate aspirin like it was candy because my back and hips hurt constantly. I had no emotions about me, and I knew at this rate I would be burned out soon.

The new year rolled around and I decided to go to Gold's Gym to see what it was all about. I met with a trainer and told him I had never been in a gym before. I also told him I had never been athletic, and he assured me not to worry. He said it would be fun. At the time, I did not see any fun in lifting weights and getting on the treadmill, but I signed up anyway.

The first week was tough on me. I was running on the treadmill in $10 Kmart shoes, and they raised blisters the size of golf balls on my feet. I knew there would be other obstacles to overcome, and the blisters were just one of them.

The second week I started the 3-Apple-a-Day GI Diet. I always hated the word "diet" because I had been on so many. But eating real food, six times a day, plus one gallon of water, felt good. This was a good plan for me. However, it was challenging when my wife and kids ordered pizza that first Friday. But I wasn't going to sacrifice the 3 pounds I had lost that week to pizza, so I settled for turkey and rice.

The fourth week, the alarm went off at 5 A.M. I sat up and noticed that the morning was different. I felt good. I slept through the night and felt laughter and happiness. I wanted to go to the gym . . . I needed my exercise now!

The day came that I will never forget. The guys in the locker room noticed I'd lost a lot of weight and encouraged me to keep it up. That made me feel good. My energy level was in overdrive and the harder I worked, the better I felt. The better I felt, the harder I worked. From that day on, my feeling toward myself and people had changed. I had a love for the gym and the people around me.

Now I get up at 5 A.M., prepare my food for the day, go to the gym, and then to work—and enjoy it! I come home from work, cook dinner, take my son to baseball, return home, and do homework with the kids. I then finish my work, visit with my family, and head to bed at 10 P.M. My energy level is always very positive and high!

I took first place in the Gold's Gym Get-in-Shape Contest, losing 47 pounds and 19 per cent body fat!

Pete won first place and $5,000, in Gold's Gym of Wenatchee's local contest, 2000, and fourth place in the national Gold's Gym Challenge, 2003.

Sandi Anderson, age 54

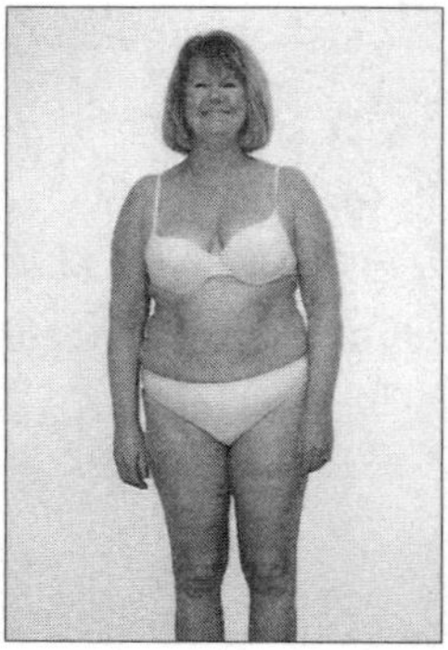

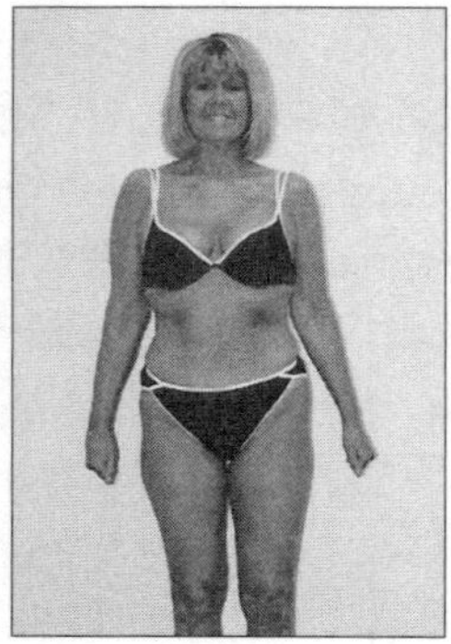

	Before	**After**	***Change***
Weight (pounds)	198	169	−29
Body fat (per cent)	41	34	−7
Waist (inches)	39.5	34.75	−4.75
Hips (inches)	43.25	40.75	−2.75
Thigh (inches)	26.75	24.25	−2.5

"You just have a slow metabolism." "It's simple, take in less calories, exercise more." "You're over 50, you're not expected to be in shape."

These are just a few of the so-called facts of life I have listened to my entire life. I have been told by many that my metabolism is slow, and I believed them. Guess what? I now know the truth. I have an above-average metabolism, and all these years my body thought it was starving!

As for taking in less calories and exercising more, what a vicious circle that is. I would start an exercise program and diet, cutting calories to less than half of the required fuel just to function through a normal day. After a few days, I was so exhausted I cut out the exercise, and of course then I had to cut out some more calories to compensate! I lost weight, but felt awful and *always* gained it back!

After seeing results from past contestants, I decided that if they could do it so could I! To the shock of many people, I decided to go for it. I have learned so much about myself in 12 weeks. I learned how my body works; why I have fought my weight my whole life; and how to maintain a healthy, fit body. This is what I have been searching for.

The 3-Apple-a-Day GI Diet was so easy to follow. I was never hungry. In fact, I had to retrain myself to eat enough. Never tiring of three apples a day, I had no cravings for sweets—I believe the Fuji apples helped in this area. I looked forward to having my apple as a snack every evening! I had more energy and was amazed at how steadily I lost weight. I plan to continue using the 3-Apple-a-Day GI Diet to maintain my weight.

I am so proud of myself! I hope I can motivate another "50 something"-year-old to take charge and be the best he or she can!

Just a small note. Before I started the challenge, I was suffering from hot flushes day and night. I now have virtually stopped them completely! It's wonderful to be free from that!

Sandi won first place and $2,200 in Gold's Gym of Wenatchee's local contest, 2003.

Donald Housden, age 55

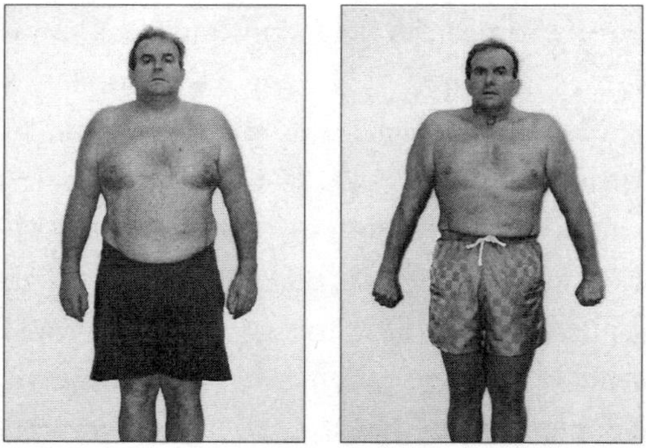

	Before	After	*Change*
Weight (pounds)	235	201	−34
Body fat (per cent)	35	26	−9
Waist (inches)	48.5	41.25	−7.25
Hips (inches)	49.25	43.5	−5.75
Thigh (inches)	24	22.75	−1.75

It was easy to rationalize my obese body when I was spammed by hundreds of TV and radio ads daily helping me feed my food addiction. I had been overweight and out of shape for years and accepted life as it was. I was comfortable and in total denial of my "non-existent" problem. You would think at 235 pounds, with shortness of breath and Type 2 diabetes, I would have a clue!

My wake-up call was when my doctor told me after my blood tests that he could no longer help me—I had to help myself. What a concept! I was to be accountable for my own fate. The way I was doing things now had to change, or else.

I know that to be good at what you do you have to practice. So I started practising being an athlete in training. I started a food journal, joined the gym, and went daily, aggressively training at being an athlete. I bought athletic clothes, so I could look like an athlete, and I would change into them as soon as I got home from work. I even wore them on my days off so I could feel like an athlete. So what if I looked like the Pillsbury Doughboy®—in my mind, I was an athlete.

The third week in the program, I had my blood work done again. My doctor thought the lab had sent the wrong results because of such drastic changes. My cholesterol had been 361; now it was 140. My triglycerides had been 721; now they were at 117. My risk factor for cholesterol fractions fell from 6.2 to 2.6. The best results were from my glucose meter, which started at a high of 445 and now was running in the 90 range *without medication!* I knew then I was on the right track!

I started to train even harder after the test results. I brushed off my bicycle, bought a stopwatch, and started riding like an athlete—setting goals and counting my spins per minute. I now ride my bike to the gym, making a round trip of 11 miles and I love it!

During my seventh week of training, we had an attempted robbery early one morning at work—a really bad person tried to duct-tape our bookkeeper and rob the safe. The bookkeeper screamed, and at first I thought she had seen a spider. But when she screamed the second time I leaped from the cash register and ran towards the office. I saw a person dressed in black running from the office. You have two seconds to make a judgement call. I, with the help of another employee, captured the robber and called the police. I felt like the guy on the Gold's Gym mural (a buffed athlete). I realized I was no longer an athlete in training; I had become an athlete.

I have just begun. I have set new goals and have new challenges to meet. I have my youth back, and my life has been restored. I will continue on this journey.

Donald won the "Most Inspirational" Award and a new mountain bike in Gold's Gym of Wenatchee's local contest, 2003.

West Mathison, age 26

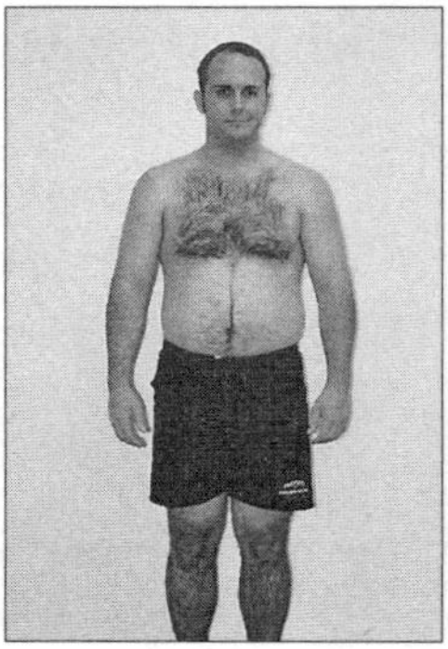

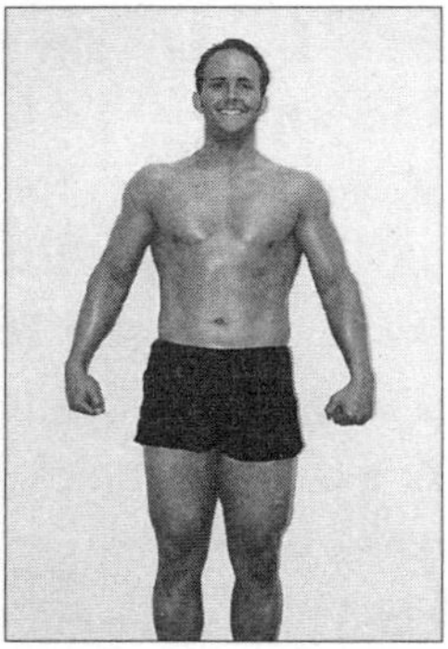

	Before	After	*Changes*
Weight (pounds)	217	185	−32
Body fat (per cent)	22	11	−11
Waist (inches)	40.5	34.25	−6.25
Hips (inches)	44.25	39.75	−4.75
Thigh (inches)	26.25	24	−2.25

TIPS ON APPLES AND TRAVELLING

During the contest, I travelled all but three weeks and was typically gone three days a week. Plus, I wasn't in a position to stop by a grocery store. Therefore, I had a little strategy to keep me consistent. Giving myself choices and keeping variety in my diet helped me stay consistent.

I'd line the bottom of my briefcase with three apples for my day of travel. During in-flight meals or at customer dinners, I'd pull an apple out of my briefcase just before eating or as we'd walk into the restaurant. My variety selection was based on the characteristics of the apples. The Cameo, Granny Smith, Red Delicious, and Pink Lady travelled best because they hold a better crunch at room temperature.

While I was away from home, I would pack (cold) refrigerated apples in my briefcase to be eaten once I arrived at my office. I would pack either Golden Delicious or Galas to refrigerate at my office. These types of apples have a thin skin and are more sensitive to warm temperatures and bruising. They too can travel, but they need protection. While they were still cold, I would put them in a sock (a clean sock!) and pack them in my suitcase. They would usually keep cool until the end of the day.

If I was at home or at the office, I'd slice an apple and use spices like chilli powder, cinnamon, and/or allspice to further the variety in my diet.

For me, having variety and being creative kept me consistent with my food plan. I did not get bored with eating apples. With all the new varieties available, I had one for any mood. Having choices made the plan seem unlimited and unregimented.

West won second place and $1,525 in Gold's Gym of Wenatchee's local contest, 2003.

PART VI

PUTTING IT ALL TOGETHER

QUICK START

You've read the book, you've heard the recommendations, and you believe the 3-Apple-a-Day GI Diet is right for you. Now, are you ready to get started on your journey to permanent fat loss?

If so, congratulations! Here are the steps to get you going. Also, check out the FAQs on page 124.

Step 1: Set your goal(s). Maybe you have one main goal, but also set mini-goals to achieve your main goal.

Step 2: Determine your calorie needs. Start with 10 calories per pound of body weight. (For example, 150 pounds × 10 = 1,500 calories.)

Step 3: Decide if you want to use the entire seven-day meal plan or just one or two days. Find your appropriate calorie level.

Step 4: Buy your food for the week. Prepare some of your meals in advance and freeze them.

Step 5: Take your measurements and/or your pictures.

Step 6: Start your exercise program (see Exercise Guidelines for Fat Loss on page 85 and 12-Week Beginner's Exercise Program on page 89).

Step 7: Begin journaling (be sure to record your food intake and track your exercise).

Step 8: Stay focused and measure your progress every two weeks.

Step 9: Ask for support from family and friends.

Step 10: *Have fun!*

Tips for Achieving the Steps

Step 1: Goals will help you keep on track and stay focused. Set mini-goals such as adding apples to your current diet each day. Turn to page 27 for more on setting your goals and creating a Personal Contract.

Step 2: When determining your calorie intake, keep in mind your current activity level. The more active you are, the more likely you'll need additional calories. For instance, if you have a desk job, you may not need as many calories as someone who works in construction. I suggest starting with 10 calories per pound of your current body weight. If you find yourself very hungry, then increase your intake by 100 calories (for example, add three quarters cup of oatmeal, one slice of turkey, or two cups of vegetables). You can find your calorie level in the Nutrient Chart for Fat Loss on page 62.

Step 3: When using the meal plans starting on page 134, some people like variety and use the full seven days. I also have clients who like simplicity, so they may use the suggested menus on only one or two days.

Step 4: Try to purchase your food and plan your meals ahead of time to prevent making poor choices when you allow yourself to become hungry. You may find planning your food for the day will give you better control over your appetite. Many of the recipes are large volume (such as Sizzlin' Grilled Chicken Breast, page 176); you can cook them up and store and/or freeze them to have food on hand so you won't have to make poor choices. Also, carry apples with you—again, to prevent those dips in blood sugar that may cause you to make poor choices.

Step 5: Taking measurements, such as at your waist and hips, every two weeks may help you see some changes that you may not notice in the mirror or on the scales. I suggest keeping a small spiral notebook to record the changes. Use the sample chart on page 15 for guidance. Also, taking pictures of yourself before you start the plan and then again four weeks later may show changes you may not otherwise notice. In the back of the book, there are pages on which you can paste your before-and-after photos.

Step 6: Increasing your activity level either through an established plan (see Chapter 15) or other physical activities will rev up your metabolism. All physical activity counts towards improving your health, whether it's doing household chores or working with a personal trainer. If you are currently inactive, try using a pedometer (available at department or sport shops) to measure how many steps you take in one day. Studies have shown that individuals who are at a healthy weight take at least 10,000 steps per day.

Step 7: Journaling your food, beverage, and physical activity habits may seem cumbersome, but studies show long-term weight management is achieved by those that continue to journal (see page 30). Make copies of the blank Food and Beverage Record form (page 219) and Weekly Exercise Tracking sheet (page 220) and record your progress. This information may come in handy later to reflect on your accomplishments.

Step 8: If you can visualize your end result (such as how you will look in your old Levi's™), it will be easier to achieve your goal. Again, take mini-steps (setting daily goals, such as exercise) to get there. Focus on achieving your daily goals, and you'll be surprised how easily the weight comes off! As mentioned in step 5, take your girth measurements every two weeks.

Step 9: Everyone needs support when taking on difficult challenges. Changing food and activity habits can be challenging and overwhelming, but the 3-Apple-a-Day GI Diet will provide the guidance you need. Find support from family, friends, or co-workers—especially if you find yourself struggling to stay on track with your newly established healthy habits. When you make a Personal Contract (page 29), you'll choose one special support person who will vow to keep you on track.

Step 10: Seriously, have fun feeling healthy and more energetic than you could have ever imagined!

THE PRE-PLAN BUILDUP

Feeling overwhelmed?

Try easing into the plan by taking one step at a time through five phases. To start, think about what you'd like to achieve. Is your goal to improve appearance, health, and/or physical fitness (see Chapter 5)?

PHASE 1, WEEK 1

To figure out what changes are needed to improve your behaviours, make a point of writing down what you do throughout your day. Be specific and include as much as you can. You can also narrate this information into a small tape recorder.

After you have completed a couple of days, make two columns: one column for food and beverages and the other for activity. Incorporate the events of your previous days in these columns and continue to do so on a daily basis from then on.

PHASE 2, WEEKS 2–3

Look at your columns of information and decide what you want to work on more—food/beverage intake or activity.

To improve your eating habits, start by simply drinking more water this week. Gradually increase the amount by one cup to reach your suggested amount (see Nutrient Chart for Fat Loss on page 62).

For activity, find 10 minutes in your day and start walking (in or out of your house) or playing with your kids or doing chores—simply moving. Dedicate these 10 minutes every day just to becoming more active.

PHASE 3, WEEKS 3–8

Food. Look at how many times you eat fruits and vegetables in the course of a day. If none, it may take a while to reach the recommended amount. Again, start small—add one apple a day each week. By three weeks, you will be up to three apples per day. Include vegetables in the evenings also. Within four to five weeks, you will be up to the nine suggested servings of fruits and vegetables.

Activity. Now is the time to add some weight training. Your recent activity has conditioned your joints, and it's time to work the muscles to help increase your bone density and metabolism. You can do it from home—get an exercise video or a good home training guide (such as *Body for Life*). You may consider finding a health club. A good health club can help guide you and ensure that you perform the exercises safely.

PHASE 4, WEEKS 9–12

Food. Now let's look at your carbohydrate intake. Carbohydrates come from breads, cereals, crackers, pasta, rice, fruits, vegetables, and more. Do you consume large quantities of these? Are carbohydrates (excluding fruits and vegetables) the main food you eat—either snacking or during a meal? (See my discussion of emotional triggers on page 33.) If so, you'll want to start including more protein. Protein foods, such as lean meats, poultry, fish, and lowfat dairy products (yogurt, milk, cheese) will help keep your blood sugar stable so you won't keep eating more and more carbohydrates. This will take some planning and thought. Look at your columns and determine how many times you are eating protein and how many times you are eating carbohydrates. Try balancing these foods.

Activity. You are on your way to a leaner, healthier body. Try out a variety of activities such as biking, power walking, aerobic class, or videos. Maybe even consider training for a special event, such as a fun-run or walkathon.

FINAL PHASE—FROM NOW ON

If you are seeing and feeling a difference, keep doing what you have been doing! You are ready for the next step, the 3-Apple-a-Day GI Diet. You have laid your foundation and will start to make real progress.

Maintaining your ideal weight

Once you have reached your goal weight, you'll want to switch to a maintenance program. In your maintenance program, your food choices will be the same, but you will need to increase your calories so you can *maintain* your ideal weight and not lose more. Your activity level should remain the same.

Maintaining will still take effort. "Maintenance" means balancing your caloric intake with your energy expenditure. The 3-Apple-a-Day GI Diet suggests that you consume 10 calories per pound of body weight daily (page 61) for fat loss. For maintenance, I recommend 12 calories per pound of body weight daily, depending on your activity levels. Remember, for good health, you should be active at least one hour per day. See page 71 for tips from clients who have been successful in maintaining their weight loss.

FAQs for the 3-Apple-a-Day GI Diet

1. **What is the 3-Apple-a-Day GI Diet?**

   Originally, it was a simple suggestion of eating an apple before each major meal to increase produce consumption and fibre intake. Later it was combined with a balanced meal plan that has proven successful for thousands in achieving permanent fat loss.

2. **How do apples work in fat loss?**

   There are several ways that apples aid in fat loss. Not only are apples packed with essential vitamins and minerals but they also provide a high amount of fibre and when eaten before meals, fill you up so you will eat less. Apples are crunchy and sweet and help curb the "sweet tooth". Apples also are very convenient to carry wherever you go, so if you're traveling in the car, they are a handy snack to tide you over until you can eat a meal, preventing you from making unhealthy quick-stop choices.

3. **Can other fruits, apple juice, or applesauce, be substituted?**

   We feature apples not only because of their "convenience" but also because of their nutrient value and low GI ranking. Not many fruits can measure up to what apples provide. In the original food plan, there were other fruits listed, with only one apple per day. It wasn't until we started suggesting three apples per day, prior to each meal, that we started seeing record fat-loss numbers in our local Get-in-Shape Contest.

4. **Why is it more difficult to lose weight now than when I was younger?**

   It really all depends on how you lost weight in the past. If you lost weight by cutting your calories way down, as most people do, and not exercising, then you probably lost some muscle tissue along the way. Muscle tissue is what keeps metabolism high and, in turn, keeps body fat low. In addition, as you age, if you don't use your muscle you'll lose it (it shrinks), resulting in an even lower metabolism. So in a nutshell, yo-yo dieting strips away your muscle tissue, makes your body hang on to your fat, and makes it extremely difficult to lose weight as you get older.

5. **My friend and I weigh the same, but she can wear two sizes smaller.**
   Your friend likely has a lower body fat and higher muscle tissue ratio than you do. Muscle is much heavier than fat, but it takes up a lot less space.
6. **Why does it seem easier for men to lose weight faster than women?**
   Men normally have higher metabolic rates because they have more muscle mass compared to women. The more muscle tissue you have, the more calories you'll burn. So ladies, you can speed up your fat loss by increasing your muscle mass—through weight training.
7. **I have a hard time drinking water. Why is it necessary?**
   Water has many functions. The most important functions for fat loss are keeping the kidneys flushed, carrying water-soluble vitamins, and keeping you feeling full.
8. **Why are high-protein, low-carb diets so popular?**
   They seem to be popular because of the quick weight-loss effect. Our society wants instant gratification, and this type of diet may provide that. Be careful, though. I've had clients try these types of diets and not only have they ended up losing valuable muscle tissue but they have also actually gained body fat! These diets are also difficult to stick with long term and may be too low in fibre for a healthy gut. Make sure you are eating five to nine servings of fruits and vegetables every day on this type of diet.
9. **Why do they say "diets don't work"?**
   Diet alone is not enough to permanently change your metabolism. "Diets" are only (usually) a quick fix and are strongly associated with deprivation. Many diets set people up for temporary weight loss but are often too restrictive or complicated to follow long term. People end up getting frustrated, or they have difficulty seeing results and stop doing the dieting.

10. **What is the difference between "good" fats and "bad" fats?**
"Good" fats, such as unsaturated fats (plant oils, fish oil, nuts), are associated with health and prevention of diseases. "Bad" fats, such as trans-fatty acids and saturated fats, are just the opposite—they are associated with disease. In fat loss, fat is fat—even good fat is fat. It doesn't take much effort to store excess dietary fat. The 3-Apple-a-Day GI Diet recommends that your fat intake be around 20 per cent of your calories. When you consume fat, try to make sure it's from an unsaturated source and in its original form (e.g., flaxseeds, not flaxseed oil).
11. **How can I avoid losing muscle tissue when I'm on a weight-loss program?**
There are three things that will help: (1) Make sure you are eating enough calories, starting with 10 calories per pound of body weight; (2) balance your carbohydrates and protein as in the 3-Apple-a-Day GI Diet; and (3) stress your muscles through weight training to make them more metabolically active.
12. **I hear a lot about "good" carbs and "bad" carbs. What's the difference?**
"Good" or "bad" carbs may be distinguished based on their rating on the Glycaemic Index. Good carbs, such as apples, have a low number. A bad carb, such as white bread or refined foods, has a high number. In simple terms, when carbs have a high GI rating and are eaten alone (not combined with a low-GI food), they tend to be easily stored as fat, thus making us even fatter.
13. **What does the term "impact carbs" or "net carbs" refer to on food packages?**
This is another marketing ploy for people on low-carb diets. This measure is derived from taking the total amount of carbs and subtracting the dietary fibre and sugar alcohols. Be wary of this marketing hook—manufacturers often take out the carbs but add fat. Therefore the number of calories may remain the same or even be higher!

PART VII

MEAL PLANS AND RECIPES

EATING AND COOKING WITH THE 3-APPLE-A-DAY GI DIET

The 3-Apple-a-Day GI Diet features seven days of planned meals tailored to your specific needs (one diet does not fit all). There are six levels starting at 1,200 and continuing to 2,500 calories.

The breakfast contains high-fibre carbohydrates and protein to raise and maintain your energy levels through the day. At the end of the day, your last meal is higher in protein and lower in carbohydrates to allow your body to rest at night. Once you reach your goal and are ready for maintenance, you can add more carbohydrates to your evening meal. But for now, keep it "light at night".

Refer to Nutrient Chart for Fat Loss (on page 62) to determine your starting calorie and nutrient levels.

More than 100 delicious recipes to choose from!

You will not feel deprived on the 3-Apple-a-Day GI Diet. You will find satisfying main courses, delicious entrées, hearty breakfast items, healthy snacks, and much more. Each recipe provides a per-serving breakdown of calories, protein, carbohydrates, fat, fibre, and sodium.

That means you won't have to wonder at the end of the day if you have consumed your 40/40/20 (40 per cent protein, 40 per cent carbohydrates, 20 per cent fat) recommendation. Or wonder if you spiked your blood sugar into orbit with high-GI foods that went right to your hips—since almost all the recipes in the meal plans are made up of low-GI ingredients. Because of the variety of food choices, some of the meal plans will vary slightly in protein, carbohydrates, and fat from the 40/40/20 recommendation.

If the recipe is provided in the book, its page number is given in the meal plan. Because calorie needs vary, make sure you check your menu to see if there are additional serving suggestions or additions to your recipe.

You may notice that some of the meals do not have an apple listed separately. These meals include dishes that contain apples in them.

Large-volume recipes

You'll find several recipes termed "large-volume recipe", which may help you prepare food ahead of time so you will have meals on hand. I suggest trying a few of these recipes and storing them in your refrigerator or freezer for later reheating. Many of the recipes freeze nicely. You can freeze food in freezer bags or plastic freezing containers. To ensure the quality and safety of the food, make sure the food has cooled before placing it in the freezer.

Glycaemic Index ranges

In the substitution list, most of the carbohydrate-containing foods have a GI number listed (see Chapter 7).

Variety is the spice of life—or not!

If you like variety in your meals, the meal plans offer seven different daily menus to satisfy those fickle taste buds. If your daily routine is busy and you prefer the simplicity of following the same one-day meal plan throughout the week, that's perfectly acceptable, too.

For added interest, you may even want to mix and match the meals from different days or use the Substitution List (page 157) to create your own meals.

Create your own daily meal plan

You also have the option of creating your own meal plan. Simply follow the meal plan guidelines in the section titled "Create Your Own". This takes more planning, of course, but you will benefit from learning how to balance your own food and make healthier choices.

Create your own recipes

Eating healthy doesn't have to be bland and boring. You can create your own tasty, exciting recipes from your own favourites, many of which can be made over to create a healthier meal. So you don't have to give up the foods you love. Several of the recipes in this book were created by people who have followed the plan.

Simply exchange some of the less-healthy ingredients in your recipes, such as oils and saturated fats, with items and foods found in the Substitution List. Your cooking will not only be healthier but will be adventurous!

Who ever said playing with your food was a bad thing?

Shopping list made simple

Your shopping list should contain the items needed for the recipes and foods in your meal plan. The amount needed will vary depending on your calorie level. Be sure to check your weekly menu to determine how much of each item you'll need.

You'll notice that the Shopping List (page 155) is divided into two categories: Weekly Groceries and Pantry Staples. Many people will have some of the pantry staples already on hand. You may consider making a photocopy of the Shopping List so you can tick off which items you already have and/or put quantities next to the items you need. Or you may just write your list on a separate sheet of paper.

Note: The Shopping List only contains foods that appear on your weekly menu. There are more than 100 recipes in this book, other than the recipes used in your plan, which you may try as well. Be sure to check the ingredients in each recipe to see if it's already on the shopping list. If not, add it before going to the shops.

If you are cooking for your family or other people using your meal plan, add the additional amount of each item you will need. For example, if you are making Salmon Caesar Salad (page 202) for four, you'll need to plan for the three extra servings. Many of the recipes make multiple servings, but you should double-check just to be sure.

How to use the Substitution List

First, find the food you want to replace in the meal plan. Then find it listed in the Substitution List (page 157) and make an exchange with another preferred choice within that category. For example, if you do not eat beef, exchange the same quantity for chicken breast (or whatever you like). Try to match the calories and protein.

Other Healthy Tips to Boost Nutrition

Item	Instead of	Try
Coffee	Cream and sugar	Skimmed milk and protein powder
In baked goods	Butter and oil	Applesauce or apple butter
	White flour	Use one-half whole-wheat flour
	Instant oatmeal	Old-fashioned porridge oats
	Sugar	Sugar substitute
	Full amount of nuts	Half the amount
Dairy products	Full fat	Low-fat or skimmed
	Whole egg	Two egg whites
Stir-fry or sauté	Oil	Cooking spray or broth
Salad dressing	Regular, full fat	Light or non-fat
Meats	Regular minced beef	7 per cent fat or less

Meal Plans

1,200-CALORIE MEAL PLAN

Create Your Own

BREAKFAST
Protein—20 grams
Carbohydrates—30 grams
Fat—5 grams

SNACK
Protein—20 grams
Carbohydrates—25 grams

LUNCH
Vegetable
Protein—30 grams
Carbohydrates—30 grams
Fat—5 grams

SNACK
Protein—20 grams
Carbohydrates—25 grams

DINNER
Carbohydrates—20 grams
Vegetables × 2
Protein—30 grams
Fat—5 grams

Calories:	1,200
Protein:	120 grams (40%)
Carbs:	120 grams (40%)
Fat:	27 grams (20%)
Fibre:	25 grams
Sodium:	2,000 mg

Day 1*

BREAKFAST
Apple
Scrambled Eggs with Salsa (page 168)
1½ ounces cooked porridge oats

SNACK
4 ounces non-fat cottage cheese

LUNCH
Apple
Sizzlin' Grilled Chicken Breast (page 176)
3 ounces steamed broccoli
Tasty Brown Rice (page 192) ¼ serving

SNACK
Cappuccino Shake (page 173)

DINNER
Grilled Salmon Salad (page 201)

Calories:	1,235
Protein:	128 grams (41%)
Carbs:	128 grams (41%)
Fat:	23 grams (17%)
Fibre:	23 grams
Sodium:	2,349 mg

**Throughout daily meal plan, use 1 serving unless noted otherwise.*

1,200-CALORIE MEAL PLAN

Day 2

BREAKFAST

Apple
Cheese Omelet (page 166)

SNACK

8 ounces non-fat yogurt

LUNCH

Apple
Turkey Salsa Burgers (page 180)
1 ounce non-fat sliced cheese
3 ounces steamed asparagus

SNACK

Strawberry Shake (page 170)

DINNER

Apple
Chicken–Broccoli Salad (page 198)

Calories:	1,205
Protein:	116 grams (39%)
Carbs:	140 grams (45%)
Fat:	22 grams (16%)
Fibre:	25 grams
Sodium:	2,733 grams

Day 3

BREAKFAST

Gourmet Oatmeal (page 160)

SNACK

Banana Strawberry Smoothie
(page 208) ½ serving

LUNCH

Apple
Turkey Lasagne (page 186)
6 ounces tossed green salad
2 tablespoons non-fat dressing

SNACK

Mocha Shake (page 173)

DINNER

Chicken Apple Stir-Fry (page 193)

Calories:	1,248
Protein:	113 grams (35%)
Carbs:	187 grams (58%)
Fat:	9 grams (7%)
Fibre:	33 grams
Sodium:	1,605 mg

1,200-CALORIE MEAL PLAN

Day 4

BREAKFAST
Apple
3 ounces high-fibre cereal
4 ounces skimmed milk

SNACK
1 celery stalk
1 tablespoon peanut butter

LUNCH
Apple
Beef Stew (page 188)

SNACK
Banana Cream Shake (page 170)

DINNER
Apple
Tuna–Mixed Green Salad (page 201)

Calories:	1,229
Protein:	114 grams (36%)
Carbs:	164 grams (52%)
Fat:	16 grams (12%)
Fibre:	32 grams
Sodium:	1,627 mg

Day 5

BREAKFAST
Apple
Cheesy Asparagus Omelet (page 167)

SNACK
Cottage Cheese and Yogurt Mix (page 205)

LUNCH
Apple
Spaghetti Sauce (page 185)
2 ounces whole-wheat pasta

SNACK
Chocolate Shake (page 169)

DINNER
Apple
Salmon Caesar Salad (page 202)

Calories:	1,209
Protein:	116 grams (38%)
Carbs:	138 grams (46%)
Fat:	22 grams (16%)
Fibre:	22 grams
Sodium:	2,419 mg

1,200-CALORIE MEAL PLAN

Day 6

BREAKFAST
Apple
Tortilla and Eggs (page 168)

SNACK
8 ounces non-fat yogurt

LUNCH
Apple
Hearty Chilli (page 187)

SNACK
Strawberry–Banana Shake (page 171)

DINNER
Waldorf Salad (page 198)

Calories:	1,304
Protein:	119 grams (36%)
Carbs:	180 grams (54%)
Fat:	15 grams (10%)
Fibre:	27 grams
Sodium:	2,630 mg

Day 7

BREAKFAST-BRUNCH
Apple slices
Fat-Free Cinnamon Rolls (page 209)
Devilled Eggs (page 169) 2 halves

SNACK
Salmon Crackers (page 204)

LUNCH
Apple
Turkey Rice Mix (page 191)
3 ounces steamed broccoli

SNACK
French Vanilla Shake (page 171)

DINNER
Taco Salad (page 201)

DESSERT
Mock Apple Pie (page 215)

Calories:	1,349
Protein:	114 grams (34%)
Carbs:	187 grams (56%)
Fat:	16 grams (10%)
Fibre:	26 grams
Sodium:	1,020 mg

1,200-CALORIE MEAL PLAN

Create Your Own

BREAKFAST
Protein—30 grams
Carbohydrates—30 grams
Fat—8 grams

SNACK
Protein—30 grams
Carbohydrates—30 grams

LUNCH
Vegetable
Protein—30 grams
Carbohydrates—40 grams
Fat—8 grams

SNACK
Protein—30 grams
Carbohydrates—30 grams

DINNER
Carbohydrates—20 grams
Vegetables × 2
Protein—30 grams
Fat—8 grams

Calories:	1,500
Protein:	150 grams (40%)
Carbs:	150 grams (40%)
Fat:	33 grams (20%)
Fibre:	25 grams
Sodium:	2,000 mg

Day 1*

BREAKFAST
Apple
Scrambled Eggs with Salsa
(page 168)
1½ ounces cooked porridge oats

SNACK
4 ounces non-fat cottage cheese

LUNCH
Apple
Sizzlin' Grilled Chicken Breast
(page 176)
3 ounces steamed broccoli
Tasty Brown Rice (page 192) ¼ serving

SNACK
Cappuccino Shake (page 173)

DINNER
Grilled Salmon Salad (page 201)
(6 ounces salmon)

Calories:	1,570
Protein:	158 grams (40%)
Carbs:	156 grams (40%)
Fat:	35 grams (20%)
Fibre:	26 grams
Sodium:	2,751 mg

**Throughout daily meal plan, use 1 serving unless noted otherwise.*

1,500-CALORIE MEAL PLAN

Day 2

BREAKFAST

Apple
Ham and Cheese Omelet (page 167)

SNACK

8 ounces non-fat yogurt

LUNCH

Apple
Turkey Salsa Burgers (page 180)
1 ounce non-fat sliced cheese
3 ounces steamed asparagus

SNACK

Strawberry Shake (page 170)

DINNER

Apple
Chicken–Broccoli Salad (page 198)

Calories:	1,498
Protein:	178 grams (46%)
Carbs:	140 grams (37%)
Fat:	28 grams (17%)
Fibre:	25 grams
Sodium:	3,643 mg

Day 3

BREAKFAST

Gourmet Oatmeal (page 160)

SNACK

Banana–Strawberry Smoothie (page 208)

LUNCH

Apple
Turkey Lasagne (page 186)
6 ounces tossed green salad
2 tablespoons non-fat dressing

SNACK

Mocha Shake (page 173)

DINNER

Chicken Apple Stir-Fry (page 193)

Calories:	1,510
Protein:	124 grams (32%)
Carbs:	232 grams (59%)
Fat:	15 grams (9%)
Fibre:	40 grams
Sodium:	1,700 mg

1,500-CALORIE MEAL PLAN

Day 4

BREAKFAST
Apple
3 ounces high-fibre cereal
4 fl. ounces skimmed milk

SNACK
1 celery stalk
2 tablespoons peanut butter

LUNCH
Apple
Beef Stew (page 188)

SNACK
Banana Cream Shake (page 170)

DINNER
Apple
Tuna–Mixed Green Salad (page 201)

Calories:	1,497
Protein:	145 grams (38%)
Carbs:	179 grams (47%)
Fat:	24 grams (15%)
Fibre:	34 grams
Sodium:	1,760 mg

Day 5

BREAKFAST
Apple
Cheesy Asparagus Omelet (page 167)
(2 ounces cheese)

SNACK
Cottage Cheese and Yogurt Mix
(page 205)

LUNCH
Apple
Spaghetti Sauce (page 185)
2 ounces whole-wheat pasta

SNACK
Chocolate Shake (page 169)

DINNER
Apple
Salmon Caesar Salad (page 202)
(6 ounces salmon)

Calories:	1,463
Protein:	149 grams (41%)
Carbs:	144 grams (39%)
Fat:	33 grams (20%)
Fibre:	22 grams
Sodium:	3,150 mg

1,500-CALORIE MEAL PLAN

Day 6

BREAKFAST
Apple
Tortilla and Eggs (page 168)

SNACK
8 ounces non-fat yogurt

LUNCH
Apple
Hearty Chilli (page 187)

SNACK
Strawberry–Banana Shake (page 171)

DINNER
Waldorf Salad (page 198)
(6 ounces chicken; 1 tablespoon nuts)

Calories:	1,536
Protein:	148 grams (38%)
Carbs:	187 grams (48%)
Fat:	25 grams (14%)
Fibre:	29 grams
Sodium:	2,891 mg

Day 7

BREAKFAST-BRUNCH
Apple slices
Fat-Free Cinnamon Rolls (page 208)
Devilled Eggs (page 169) 3 halves

SNACK
Salmon Crackers (page 204)
(2 ounces salmon)

LUNCH
Apple
Turkey Rice Mix (page 191)
3 ounces steamed broccoli

SNACK
French Vanilla Shake (page 171)

DINNER
Taco Salad (page 201)

DESSERT
Mock Apple Pie (page 215)

Calories:	1,498
Protein:	133 grams (36%)
Carbs:	188 grams (50%)
Fat:	23 grams (14%)
Fibre:	26 grams
Sodium:	1,186 mg

1,800-CALORIE MEAL PLAN

Create Your Own

BREAKFAST
Protein—36 grams
Carbohydrates—40 grams
Fat—10 grams

SNACK
Protein—36 grams
Carbohydrates—40 grams

LUNCH
Vegetable
Protein—36 grams
Carbohydrates—40 grams
Fat—10 grams

SNACK
Protein—36 grams
Carbohydrates—40 grams

DINNER
Carbohydrates—20 grams
Vegetables × 2
Protein—36 grams
Fat—10 grams

Calories:	1,800
Protein:	180 grams (40%)
Carbs:	180 grams (40%)
Fat:	40 grams (20%)
Fibre:	30 grams
Sodium:	2,500 mg

Day 1*

BREAKFAST
Apple
Scrambled Eggs with Salsa (page 168)
3 ounces cooked porridge oats

SNACK
4 ounces non-fat cottage cheese

LUNCH
Apple
Sizzlin' Grilled Chicken Breast (page 176) 1½ breasts
3 ounces steamed broccoli
Tasty Brown Rice (page 192)

SNACK
Cappuccino Shake (page 173)

DINNER
Grilled Salmon Salad (page 201)
(6 ounces salmon)

Calories:	1,824
Protein:	186 grams (41%)
Carbs:	181 grams (40%)
Fat:	38 grams (19%)
Fibre:	28 grams
Sodium:	3,285 mg

**Throughout daily meal plan, use 1 serving unless noted otherwise.*

1,800-CALORIE MEAL PLAN

Day 2

BREAKFAST
Apple
Ham and Cheese Omelet (page 167)

SNACK
8 ounces non-fat yogurt

LUNCH
Apple
Turkey Salsa Burgers (page 180)
1 whole-wheat bun
1 ounce non-fat sliced cheese
3 ounces steamed asparagus

SNACK
Strawberry Shake (page 170)

DINNER
Apple
Chicken–Broccoli Salad (page 198)
(6 ounces chicken breast)

Calories:	1,791
Protein:	213 grams (46%)
Carbs:	170 grams (37%)
Fat:	33 grams (17%)
Fibre:	31 grams
Sodium:	4,580 mg

Day 3

BREAKFAST
Gourmet Oatmeal (page 160)

SNACK
Banana–Strawberry Smoothie
(page 208)

LUNCH
Apple
Turkey Lasagne (page 186)
1½ servings
6 ounces tossed green salad
2 tablespoons non-fat dressing

SNACK
Mocha Shake (page 173)

DINNER
Chicken Apple Stir-Fry (page 193)
2 servings

Calories:	1,832
Protein:	169 grams (36%)
Carbs:	260 grams (55%)
Fat:	19 grams (9%)
Fibre:	46 grams
Sodium:	2,363 mg

1,800-CALORIE MEAL PLAN

Day 4

BREAKFAST

Apple
6 ounces high-fibre cereal
8 fl. ounces skimmed milk

SNACK

1 celery stalk
2 tablespoons peanut butter

LUNCH

Apple
Beef Stew (page 188) 2 servings

SNACK

Banana Cream Shake Deluxe (page 170)

DINNER

Apple
Tuna–Mixed Green Salad (page 201)

Calories:	1,791
Protein:	172 grams (38%)
Carbs:	218 grams (47%)
Fat:	28 grams (15%)
Fibre:	41 grams
Sodium:	2,237 mg

Day 5

BREAKFAST

Apple
Cheesy Asparagus Omelet (page 167) (2 ounces cheese)

SNACK

Cottage Cheese and Yogurt Mix (page 205) 1½ servings

LUNCH

Apple
Spaghetti Sauce (page 185) 2 servings
4 ounces whole-wheat pasta

SNACK

Chocolate Shake (page 169)

DINNER

Apple
Salmon Caesar Salad (page 202) (6 ounces salmon)

Calories:	1,795
Protein:	180 grams (40%)
Carbs:	178 grams (40%)
Fat:	40 grams (20%)
Fibre:	29 grams
Sodium:	3,850 mg

1,800-CALORIE MEAL PLAN

Day 6

BREAKFAST
Apple
Tortilla and Eggs (page 168)
2 servings

SNACK
Blueberry–Peach Smoothie
(page 208)

LUNCH
Apple
Hearty Chilli (page 187)

SNACK
Strawberry–Banana Shake (page 171)

DINNER
Waldorf Salad (page 198)
(6 ounces chicken; 1 tablespoon nuts)

Calories:	1,803
Protein:	160 grams (35%)
Carbs:	231 grams (50%)
Fat:	31 grams (15%)
Fibre:	39 grams
Sodium:	3,061 mg

Day 7

BREAKFAST-BRUNCH
Apple slices
Fat-Free Cinnamon Rolls (page 209)
Devilled Eggs (page 169) 6 halves

SNACK
Salmon Crackers (page 204)
(2 ounces salmon)

LUNCH
Apple
Turkey Rice Mix (page 191)
3 ounces steamed broccoli

SNACK
French Vanilla Shake (page 171)

DINNER
Taco Salad (page 201) 2 servings

DESSERT
Mock Apple Pie (page 215)

Calories:	1,794
Protein:	175 grams (39%)
Carbs:	196 grams (44%)
Fat:	34 grams (17%)
Fibre:	28 grams
Sodium:	1,694 mg

2,000-CALORIE MEAL PLAN

Create Your Own

BREAKFAST
Protein—40 grams
Carbohydrates—50 grams
Fat—12 grams

SNACK
Protein—40 grams
Carbohydrates—40 grams

LUNCH
Vegetable
Protein—40 grams
Carbohydrates—50 grams
Fat—12 grams

SNACK
Protein—40 grams
Carbohydrates—40 grams

DINNER
Carbohydrates—20 grams
Vegetables × 2
Protein—36 grams
Fat—12 grams

Calories:	2,000
Protein:	200 grams (40%)
Carbs:	200 grams (40%)
Fat:	44 grams (20%)
Fibre:	35 grams
Sodium:	3,000 mg

Day 1*

BREAKFAST
Apple
Scrambled Eggs with Salsa (page 168)
3 ounces cooked porridge oats

SNACK
4 ounces non-fat cottage cheese

LUNCH
Apple
Sizzlin' Grilled Chicken Breast (page 176) 1½ breasts
3 ounces steamed broccoli
Tasty Brown Rice (page 192)

SNACK
Peanut Butter Shake Deluxe (page 172)

DINNER
Grilled Salmon Salad (page 201) (6 ounces salmon)

Calories:	2,002
Protein:	191 grams (38%)
Carbs:	205 grams (41%)
Fat:	47 grams (21%)
Fibre:	32 grams
Sodium:	3,388 mg

**Throughout daily meal plan, use 1 serving unless noted otherwise.*

2,000-CALORIE MEAL PLAN

Day 2

BREAKFAST

Apple
Ham and Cheese Omelet (page 167)

SNACK

8 ounces non-fat yogurt
2 ounces lowfat muesli

LUNCH

Apple
Turkey Salsa Burgers (page 180)
2 servings
1 whole-wheat bun
1 ounce non-fat sliced cheese
3 ounces steamed asparagus

SNACK

Strawberry Shake (page 170)

DINNER

Apple
Chicken–Broccoli Salad (page 198)
(6 ounces chicken)

Calories:	1,960
Protein:	219 grams (44%)
Carbs:	205 grams (41%)
Fat:	35 grams (15%)
Fibre:	37 grams
Sodium:	4,764 mg

Day 3

BREAKFAST

Gourmet Oatmeal (page 160)
1½ servings

SNACK

Banana–Strawberry Smoothie
(page 208)

LUNCH

Apple
Turkey Lasagne (page 186)
1½ servings
6 ounces tossed green salad
2 tablespoons non-fat dressing

SNACK

Mocha Shake Deluxe (page 173)

DINNER

Chicken Apple Stir-Fry (page 193)
2 servings

Calories:	1,966
Protein:	182 grams (36%)
Carbs:	278 grams (55%)
Fat:	20 grams (9%)
Fibre:	49 grams
Sodium:	2,400 mg

2,000-CALORIE MEAL PLAN

Day 4

BREAKFAST
Apple
6 ounces high-fibre cereal
12 fl. ounces skimmed milk

SNACK
1 celery stalk
2 tablespoons peanut butter

LUNCH
Apple
Beef Stew (page 188) 2 servings

SNACK
Banana Cream Shake Deluxe
(page 170)

DINNER
Apple
Tuna–Mixed Green Salad (page 201)
(9 ounces tuna)

Calories:	2,021
Protein:	202 grams (39%)
Carbs:	232 grams (45%)
Fat:	36 grams (16%)
Fibre:	45 grams
Sodium:	2,793 mg

Day 5

BREAKFAST
Apple
Cheesy Asparagus Omelet (page 167)
(2 ounces cheese)

SNACK
Cottage Cheese and Yogurt Mix
(page 205)
2 servings

LUNCH
Apple
Spaghetti Sauce (page 185)
2 servings
6 ounces whole-wheat pasta

SNACK
Chocolate Shake Deluxe (page 169)

DINNER
Apple
Salmon Caesar Salad (page 202)
(6 ounces salmon)

Calories:	1,961
Protein:	196 grams (40%)
Carbs:	204 grams (41%)
Fat:	42 grams (19%)
Fibre:	32 grams
Sodium:	4,293 mg

2,000-CALORIE MEAL PLAN

Day 6

BREAKFAST
Apple
Tortilla and Eggs (page 168)
2 servings

SNACK
Blueberry–Peach Smoothie
(page 208)

LUNCH
Apple
Hearty Chilli (page 187) 2 servings

SNACK
Strawberry–Banana Shake (page 171)

DINNER
Waldorf Salad (page 198)
(6 ounces chicken; 1 tablespoon nuts)

Calories:	2,017
Protein:	181 grams (35%)
Carbs:	263 grams (51%)
Fat:	33 grams (14%)
Fibre:	48 grams
Sodium:	3,899 mg

Day 7

BREAKFAST-BRUNCH
Apple slices
Fat-Free Cinnamon Rolls (page 209)
Devilled Eggs (page 169) 6 halves

SNACK
Salmon Crackers (page 204)
(3 ounces salmon
plus 2 ounces soft cheese)

LUNCH
Apple
Turkey Rice Mix (page 191)
1½ servings
3 ounces steamed broccoli

SNACK
French Vanilla Shake (page 171)

DINNER
Taco Salad (page 201) 2 servings

DESSERT
Mock Apple Pie (page 215)

Calories:	2,017
Protein:	199 grams (40%)
Carbs:	215 grams (43%)
Fat:	39 grams (17%)
Fibre:	28 grams
Sodium:	1,870 mg

2,500-CALORIE MEAL PLAN

Create Your Own

BREAKFAST
Protein—50 grams
Carbohydrate— 60 grams
Fat—14 grams

SNACK
Protein—50 grams
Carbohydrates—50 grams

LUNCH
Vegetable
Protein—50 grams
Carbohydrates—70 grams
Fat—14 grams

SNACK
Protein—50 grams
Carbohydrates—50 grams

DINNER
Carbohydrates—20 grams
Vegetables × 2
Protein—50 grams
Fat—14 grams

Calories:	2,500
Protein:	250 grams (40%)
Carbs:	250 grams (40%)
Fat:	56 grams (20%)
Fibre:	40 grams
Sodium:	3,000 mg

Day 1*

BREAKFAST
Apple
Scrambled Eggs with Salsa (page 168) 1½ servings
4½ ounces cooked porridge oats

SNACK
4 ounces non-fat cottage cheese
1 medium pear

LUNCH
Apple
Sizzlin' Grilled Chicken Breast 2 Servings (page 176)
3 ounces steamed broccoli
Tasty Brown Rice (page 192) 1½ servings

SNACK
Peanut Butter Shake Deluxe (page 172)

DINNER
Grilled Salmon Salad (page 201) (6 ounces salmon)

Calories:	2,488
Protein:	240 grams (39%)
Carbs:	250 grams (40%)
Fat:	59 grams (21%)
Fibre:	37 grams
Sodium:	4,248 mg

**Throughout daily meal plan, use 1 serving unless noted otherwise.*

2,500-CALORIE MEAL PLAN

Day 2

BREAKFAST
Apple
Ham and Cheese Omelet (page 167)
2 servings

SNACK
8 ounces non-fat yogurt
3 ounces low-fat muesli

LUNCH
Apple
Turkey Salsa Burgers (page 180)
2 servings
1 whole-wheat bun
1 ounce non-fat sliced cheese
3 ounces steamed asparagus

SNACK
Strawberry Shake (page 170)

DINNER
Apple
Chicken–Broccoli Salad (page 198)
(6 ounces chicken breast)

Calories:	2,456
Protein:	288 grams (46%)
Carbs:	229 grams (37%)
Fat:	48 grams (17%)
Fibre:	41 grams
Sodium:	6,956 mg

Day 3

BREAKFAST
Gourmet Oatmeal (page 160)
2 servings

SNACK
Banana–Strawberry Smoothie
(page 208)

LUNCH
Apple
Turkey Lasagne (page 186)
1½ servings
9 ounces tossed green salad
3 tablespoons non-fat dressing
2 tablespoons sliced almonds

SNACK
Mocha Shake Deluxe (page 173)

DINNER
Chicken Apple Stir-Fry (page 193)
2 servings

Calories:	2,492
Protein:	234 grams (37%)
Carbs:	332 grams (52%)
Fat:	31 grams (11%)
Fibre:	57 grams
Sodium:	3,095 mg

2,500-CALORIE MEAL PLAN

Day 4

BREAKFAST
8 ounces high-fibre cereal
12 fl. ounces skimmed milk

SNACK
1 celery stalk
2 tablespoons peanut butter

LUNCH
Apple
Beef Stew (page 188) 3 servings

SNACK
Banana Cream Shake Deluxe (page 170)

DINNER
Apple
Tuna–Mixed Green Salad (page 201) (12 ounces tuna)

Calories:	2,476
Protein:	252 grams (40%)
Carbs:	285 grams (45%)
Fat:	41 grams (15%)
Fibre:	53 grams
Sodium:	3,558 mg

Day 5

BREAKFAST
Apple
Cheesy Asparagus Omelet (page 167) 2 servings

SNACK
Cottage Cheese and Yogurt Mix (page 205) 2 servings

LUNCH
Apple
Spaghetti Sauce (page 185) 2 servings
6 ounces whole-wheat pasta

SNACK
Chocolate Shake Deluxe (page 169)

DINNER
Apple
Salmon Caesar Salad (page 202) (9 ounces salmon)

Calories:	2,479
Protein:	262 grams (43%)
Carbs:	223 grams (36%)
Fat:	58 grams (21%)
Fibre:	33 grams
Sodium:	4,916 mg

2,500-CALORIE MEAL PLAN

Day 6

BREAKFAST
Apple
Tortilla and Eggs (page 168) 2 servings (plus 2 ounces non-fat cheese)

SNACK
Blueberry–Peach Smoothie (page 208)

LUNCH
Apple
Hearty Chilli (page 187) 2 servings

SNACK
Strawberry-Banana Shake Deluxe (page 171)

DINNER
Waldorf Salad (page 198) (6 ounces chicken; 1 tablespoon nuts)

Calories:	2,505
Protein:	239 grams (37%)
Carbs:	310 grams (48%)
Fat:	42 grams (15%)
Fibre:	51 grams
Sodium:	4,325 mg

Day 7

BREAKFAST-BRUNCH
Apple slices
Fat-Free Cinnamon Roll (page 209)
Devilled Eggs (page 169) 6 halves

SNACK
Salmon Crackers (page 204) (3 ounces salmon plus 2 ounces cream cheese)

LUNCH
Apple
Turkey Rice Mix (page 191) 2 servings
3 ounces steamed broccoli

SNACK
French Vanilla Shake Deluxe (page 171)

DINNER
Taco Salad (page 201) 2 servings

DESSERT
Mock Apple Pie (page 215)

Calories:	2,515
Protein:	249 grams (40%)
Carbs:	278 grams (45%)
Fat:	40 grams (15%)
Fibre:	35 grams
Sodium:	2,147 mg

THE 3-APPLE-A-DAY SHOPPING LIST

WEEKLY GROCERIES

Meats, Fish, and Poultry
Chicken breast
Turkey breast
4% lean minced beef
Flank steak
Salmon

Vegetables, Fresh
Broccoli
Cauliflower
Onion
Mushrooms
Lettuce, romaine and mixed
Spinach
Asparagus
Courgettes
Green and red peppers
Celery
Carrot
Red potatoes
Tomato
Sugar snap peas
Bean sprouts

Eggs and Dairy
Skimmed milk
Non-fat cottage cheese
Non-fat yogurt
Eggs
Egg substitute
Non-fat shredded cheddar cheese
Non-fat shredded mozzarella cheese
Non-fat sliced cheese
Non-fat cream cheese
Parmesan cheese, shredded
Light margarine

Canned Goods
Tuna, albacore
Chicken breast
Salmon
Kidney beans, low sodium
Black beans
Italian stewed tomatoes, diced
Tomato paste
Tomato sauce
Evaporated skimmed milk

Fruits, Fresh
Apples
Strawberries
Bananas
Blueberries
Peaches

Grains and Cereals
Porridge oats
High-fibre cereal, low-sodium
Spaghetti noodles, whole-wheat
Lasagne noodles
Brown or wild rice
Flour tortilla, whole-wheat
Rye Crisp crackers, fat-free
Low-fat muesli

PANTRY STAPLES

Herbs and Spices
Cinnamon
Garlic powder
Basil
Oregano
Chilli powder
Salt
Pepper
Seasoning salt
Taco seasoning

Other Items
Chicken stock cubes
Peanut butter, reduced-fat
Coffee
Buns, whole-wheat
Protein powder (soy or whey)

Baking Goods
Whole-wheat flour
Enriched white flour
Sugar
Sugar substitute (Splenda™)
Yeast
Applesauce, unsweetened
Raisins
Walnuts
Almonds
Brown sugar
Icing sugar
Vanilla flavouring

Condiments
Salsa
Rice vinegar
Soy sauce, low-sodium
Salad dressings, non-fat or light
Dijon mustard
Fat-free liquid coffee creamer, French vanilla
Worcestershire sauce
Teriyaki sauce
Non-fat mayonnaise

This shopping list is only for the foods and recipe items in the seven-day meal plans. If you are using other recipes or making substitutions, be sure you add the additional food ingredients to your weekly shopping list.

The 3-Apple-a-Day GI Diet Substitution List

Use this substitution list to replace foods in the meal plan with foods that are in the same group. For example, in the proteins, replace 3 ounces of salmon with 3 ounces of chicken breast.

		Amount	Calories	Protein (g)	Carbs (g)	Fat (g)	Fibre (g)	GI	Omega-6 Fatty Acids (g)	Omega-3 Fatty Acids (g)
Proteins	Chicken breast	3 ounces	140	26	0	3	0	—	0.4	Trace
	Turkey breast	3 ounces	114	26	0	0.6	0	—	0.27	0.01
	Extra-lean beef	3 ounces	201	26	0	10	0	—	0.3	Trace
	Tuna	3 ounces	99	22	0	0.7	0	—	0.3	0.3
	Halibut, bass, snapper	3 ounces	119	23	0	2.5	0	—	0.2	0.1
	Salmon	3 ounces	155	22	0	7	0	—	0.6	0.1
	Cod, orange roughy	3 ounces	89	20	0	0.7	0	—	Trace	Trace
	Shrimp	3 ounces	118	23	1	1.9	0	—	0.1	Trace
	Skimmed milk	8 fl. ounces	80	8	11	1	0	32	0.1	0.005
	Non-fat cottage cheese	4 ounces	121	25	3	0.6	0	—	—	—
	Non-fat yogurt	8 ounces	127	13	17	0.4	0	14	—	—
	Egg whites	6	99	21	2	0	0	—	—	—
	Kidney beans/legumes	4 ounces	163	11	29	0.6	7	27	0.3	0.6
	Light tofu	332 grams	124	21	4	2.7	0	—	0.14	0.22
	Vegetable burger	113 grams	200	10	28	5	4	—	2.3	0.14
	Whey protein powder	5 tbsp	115	20	4	2	1	—	—	—

		Amount	Calories	Protein (g)	Carbs (g)	Fat (g)	Fibre (g)	GI	Omega-6 Fatty Acids (g)	Omega-3 Fatty Acids (g)
Carbohydrates										
GRAINS	Porridge oats, cooked	3 ounces	145	6	25	2.3	5	49	0.39	0.34
	Whole-wheat hot cereal	4 ounces	133	5	28	1	4	—	—	—
	Potato, baked	202 grams	220	5	51	0.2	5	85	0.65	0.02
	Sweet potato, yam	5 ounces	158	2	38	0.2	5	54	0.08	0.016
	Brown rice	2 ounces	232	5	50	1	3	55	—	—
	Pasta, whole-wheat	4 ounces	197	7	40	1	4	37	0.28	0.14
	Cereal, shredded wheat	3 ounces	167	5	41	0.5	6	58	—	—
	Ry-Crisp, fat-free crackers	2 pieces	48	2	10	0	1.5	69	—	—
FRUIT	Apple, medium	1 each	81	0.3	21	0.5	4	38	0.12	0.025
	Banana, small	1 each	93	1	24	0.5	2	55	0.057	0.03
	Cherries	10 whole	45	1	10	0	1	22	0.1	0.1
	Apricots	3 small	50	1.5	12	0.4	2.5	57	0.081	0
	Grapefruit	1 whole	74	1.4	18	0.2	3	25	0.047	0.012
	Grapes	6 ounces	58	0.6	16	0.3	1.3	46	0.07	0.022
	Nectarine	1 medium	67	1.3	16	0.6	2	42	0.3	0.007
	Orange	1 medium	64	1	16	0	3	44	0.047	0.017
	Pear	1 small	98	0.6	25	0.6	4	38	0.15	0.002
	Peach	1 medium	42	0.6	11	0	2	42	0.043	0.001

VEGETABLES	Broccoli, raw or 1½ ounces cooked	1 cup	27	3	5	0.3	2.5	—	0.03	0.1
	Cauliflower, raw or 1½ ounces cooked	3 ounces	28	2	5	0.2	3	—	0.02	0.076
	Cabbage, raw	3 ounces	33	1.5	7	0.6	3.5	—	0.036	0.048
	Mushrooms, raw	2 ounces	18	2	3	0.2	1	—	0.128	0.001
	Spinach, raw	3 ounces	7	1	1	0	1	—	0.007	0.0035
	Courgettes, raw	2 ounces	29	1	7	0	3	—	0.025	0.042
	Asparagus, cooked	4 ounces	43	5	8	0	3	—	—	—
	French beans, cooked	3 ounces	44	2.4	10	0.3	4	—	0.07	0.11
	Carrots, raw baby	10	86	2	18.5	4	1	49	0.34	0.05
	Romaine lettuce	3 ounces	8	1	1	1	1	—	0.017	0.04
	Green leaf lettuce	3 ounces	10	0.7	2	1	0	—	0.26	0.01
Fats	Canola oil	1 tbsp	124	0	0	14	0	—	2.84	1.3
	Olive oil	1 tbsp	119	0	0	13.5	0	—	1.067	0.08
	Flaxseed oil	1 tbsp	124	0	0	14	0	—	—	—
	Flax seeds, whole	1 tbsp	59	2	4	4	3	—	0.5	2.17
	Walnuts	1 tbsp	47	2	1	4.4	0.4	—	2.61	0.25

RECIPES

BREAKFAST FOODS

Oat Cakes

Quick

6 egg whites
3 ounces porridge oats, uncooked
4 ounces non-fat cottage cheese

Beat egg whites with a fork until bubbly. Add oats and cottage cheese. Spray a deep frying pan with non-stick cooking spray and place over medium heat. Pour a bit at a time, in three spots, spacing at least 3 inches apart. Cook until golden brown. Makes 8 servings.

Optional: Top with non-fat yogurt and cooked diced apples.

Per serving without topping:
Calories: 61 *Fat: 0.3 gram*
Protein: 7 grams *Fibre: 1 gram*
Carbohydrates: 8 grams
Sodium: 114 milligrams

Gourmet Oatmeal

Quick

3 ounces cooked porridge oats
1 medium apple, cored and diced
2 tablespoons vanilla protein powder
1 teaspoon cinnamon

Mix all ingredients and enjoy! You can also cook the apples with the oatmeal. Makes 1 serving.

Calories: 252 *Fat: 1.5 grams*
Protein: 11 grams *Fibre: 9 grams*
Carbohydrates: 53 grams
Sodium: 24 milligrams

Cereal Blend

Quick

- 4 ounces high-fibre, low-sodium cereal
- 2 ounces spoon-sized shredded wheat
- 2 ounces low-fat muesli
- 8 fl. ounces skimmed milk

Mix cereals and add milk. Makes 1 serving.

Calories: 368 *Fat: 2.8 grams*
Protein: 21 grams *Fibre: 14 grams*
Carbohydrates: 77 grams
Sodium: 240 milligrams

Bran Muffins

- 3¾ ounces all-purpose flour
- 2½ ounces whole-wheat flour
- 1 tablespoon baking powder
- 2 ounces sugar
- ½ teaspoon salt
- 4 ounces 100% bran cereal
- 8 fl. ounces skimmed milk
- 2 egg whites
- 3 ounces unsweetened applesauce

Preheat oven to 400°F/200°C/GM6. Spray 12 medium muffin cups with non-stick cooking spray. Combine flours, baking powder, sugar, and salt; set aside. In a mixing bowl, combine cereal and milk; let stand for 2 minutes. Add egg whites and applesauce; mix well. Add dry ingredients, stirring just until combined. Spoon into prepared muffin cups. Bake 15 to 18 minutes or until golden brown. Serve warm. Makes 12 servings.

Optional: Add 5 ounces berries to the batter for variety.

Calories: 95 *Fat: 0*
Protein: 4 grams *Fibre: 2.4 grams*
Carbohydrates: 20 grams
Sodium: 131 milligrams

Breakfast Quesadilla

Quick

3 egg whites
1 tablespoon diced green pepper
1 tablespoon chopped onion
1 ounce non-fat shredded Cheddar cheese
2 low-fat whole-wheat tortillas
1 ounce non-fat shredded mozzarella cheese
2 tablespoons mild salsa

Use a 9-inch deep frying pan over medium heat or microwave on high in a flat baking dish (such as a pie plate) to cook eggs, pepper, onion, and Cheddar cheese. Cook flat, and flip once. Heat tortillas in microwave for 30 seconds. Place egg mixture on first tortilla and cover with the second tortilla. Sprinkle with mozzarella cheese, and top with salsa. Makes 1 serving.

Calories: 297 *Fat: 1.5 grams*
Protein: 29 grams *Fibre: 4 grams*
Carbohydrates: 53 grams
Sodium: 1401 milligrams

Breakfast Burrito

Quick

3 egg whites
1 tablespoon diced green and red peppers
1 whole-wheat tortilla
Light margarine (optional)

Cook egg whites and peppers in microwave for 1 to 2 minutes or in a small sauté pan over medium heat until eggs are cooked. Heat tortilla in microwave for 20 seconds. Lightly spread margarine on tortilla, then place eggs down the middle and roll up. Makes 1 serving.

Optional: Add non-fat cheese and/or salsa. This will add a few more calories.

Calories: 126 *Fat: 0.5 grams*
Protein: 13 grams *Fibre: 2 grams*
Carbohydrates: 23 grams
Sodium: 331 milligrams

Egg Casserole

Quick

- 12 egg whites
- 8 large mushrooms, sliced
- 2 ounces non-fat shredded cheese
- 4 tablespoons salsa

Spray microwave-safe dish with non-stick cooking spray. Cook egg substitute with mushrooms in microwave until eggs are cooked, 1 to 2 minutes. Add cheese and mix. Cook for another 45 seconds until cheese melts. Top with salsa. Makes 4 servings.

Calories: 87 *Fat: 0 gram*
Protein: 15 grams *Fibre: 0.7 grams*
Carbohydrates: 6 grams
Sodium: 424 milligrams

Breakfast in a Blender

Quick

- 6 fl. ounces non-fat milk
- 5 tablespoons protein powder (chocolate or vanilla)
- 1½ ounces oatmeal, uncooked
- 2 medium bananas
- Ice

Blend ingredients until smooth. Makes 1 serving.

Calories: 436 *Fat: 2 grams*
Protein: 38 grams *Fibre: 9 grams*
Carbohydrates: 70 grams
Sodium: 165 milligrams

Turkey Breast Sausage Patties

by Rosalie McPherson

Large-Volume Recipe

2 ounces chopped onion
2 ounces shredded and peeled apple
1 garlic clove, minced
3 teaspoons dried thyme
3 teaspoons dried, rubbed sage
1 teaspoon salt
½ teaspoon black pepper
2 pounds ground turkey breast

Spray non-stick cooking spray in deep frying pan and heat over medium-high heat. Add onion and apple; sauté for 3 minutes. Add garlic; sauté for 30 seconds. Remove onion mixture from pan; cool completely. Combine onion mixture, thyme, sage, salt, pepper, and turkey, stirring well to combine. Divide mixture into 24 equal portions, shaping each into a ½-inch-thick patty. Heat a large frying pan coated with non-stick cooking spray over medium heat. Add half of the patties; cook for 3 minutes on each side or until done. Keep warm. Repeat procedure with remaining patties. Makes 8 servings (3 patties per serving).

Calories: 156 *Fat: 3 grams*
Protein: 32 grams *Fibre: 0 gram*
Carbohydrates: 1 gram
Sodium: 74 milligrams

One-Dish Spicy Breakfast Casserole

by Nancy Van Hoven

Quick and Large-Volume Recipe

2 tablespoons chilli powder
One 32-ounce can refried beans, fat-free
Two 4-ounce cans diced green chillies
24 egg whites
6 ounces low-fat mozzarella cheese
8 ounces salsa

Preheat oven to 350°F/180°C/GM4. Mix chile powder with beans and spread in a 9 × 13 baking dish. Top with chillies, then pour egg whites over. Bake for 20 to 30 minutes, just until the eggs are set. Top with cheese then salsa. Makes 18 servings.

Calories: 76 *Fat: 1.5 grams*
Protein: 6.5 grams *Fibre: 2.4 grams*
Carbohydrates: 9 grams
Sodium: 347 milligrams

EGGS

Egg-White-Only Omelet

6 large egg whites
Salsa (optional)

Beat egg whites until large bubbles form. Spray small sauté pan or omelet pan with non-stick cooking spray. Pour in egg whites and cook over medium heat. Cook egg whites until they are white and mostly cooked. Fold the egg white circle in half, or just close the omelet pan. Top with salsa and serve. Makes 1 serving.

Calories: 99 *Fat: 0 gram*
Protein: 21 grams *Fibre: 0 gram*
Carbohydrates: 2 grams
Sodium: 298 milligrams

Basic Omelet

1 whole egg
5 egg whites
Salsa (optional)

Beat whole egg and egg whites until large bubbles form. Spray small sauté pan or omelet pan with non-stick cooking spray. Pour in eggs and cook over medium heat. Cook eggs until firm, 5 to 6 minutes. Fold the egg white circle in half, or just close the omelet pan. Top with salsa and serve. Makes 1 serving.

Calories: 161 *Fat: 5 grams*
Protein: 24 grams *Fibre: 0 gram*
Carbohydrates: 2 grams
Sodium: 335 milligrams

Cheese Omelet

Basic Omelet (above)
1 ounce non-fat Cheddar cheese

Follow directions for Basic Omelet. Sprinkle cheese in the middle, then fold the circle in half. Makes 1 serving.

Calories: 203 *Fat: 5 grams*
Protein: 30 grams *Fibre: 0 gram*
Carbohydrates: 5 grams
Sodium: 530 milligrams

Ham and Cheese Omelet

6 large egg whites plus 1 yolk
1 ounce extra lean ham
1 ounce cheese

Follow directions for Basic Omelet (page 166). Sprinkle ham and cheese in the middle, then fold the circle in half. Makes 1 serving.

Calories: 225 *Fat: 6.6 grams*
Protein: 34 grams *Fibre: 0 gram*
Carbohydrates: 5 grams
Sodium: 675 milligrams

Cheesy Asparagus Omelet

6 egg whites plus 1 yolk
4 small asparagus spears, chopped
1 ounce non-fat cheese

Follow directions for Basic Omelet (page 166). Add asparagus and cheese in the middle, then fold the circle in half. Makes 1 serving.

Calories: 217 *Fat: 5 grams*
Protein: 30 grams *Fibre: 1.3 grams*
Carbohydrates: 10 grams
Sodium: 532 milligrams

Tortilla and Eggs

3 egg whites
1 tablespoon chopped green and red peppers
1 whole-wheat tortilla
Light margarine (optional)

Cook egg whites and peppers in microwave for 1 to 2 minutes or in small sauté pan over medium heat until eggs are cooked. Heat tortilla in microwave for 20 seconds. Lightly spread margarine on tortilla, then place eggs down the middle and roll up. Makes 1 serving.

Optional: Add non-fat cheese and/or salsa. This will add a few more calories.

Calories: 126 *Fat: 0.5 gram*
Protein: 13 grams *Fibre: 2 grams*
Carbohydrates: 23 grams
Sodium: 331 milligrams

Scrambled Eggs with Salsa

6 egg whites plus 1 yolk
Chunky salsa

Beat egg whites until bubbly. Spray a microwave bowl or sauté pan with non-stick cooking spray. Cook in microwave for 45 seconds, stir. Cook another 45 to 60 seconds until eggs are cooked. Or cook in small pan over medium heat until eggs are cooked. Place on plate and top with salsa. Makes 1 to 2 servings.

Calories: 157 *Fat: 5 grams*
Protein: 24 grams *Fibre: 0 gram*
Carbohydrates: 2 grams
Sodium: 310 milligrams

Devilled Eggs

4 hard-cooked eggs
2 ounces non-fat mayonnaise
2 tablespoons Dijon or yellow mustard
½ celery stalk, diced finely
Salt (optional)
Paprika

Slice eggs in half. Save two yolks and place in a bowl. Throw away the other yolks. Set aside 6 halved egg whites. Put other egg whites in bowl with yolks. Add all other ingredients and blend. Spoon yolk mixture into egg white halves. Sprinkle with paprika. Refrigerate. Makes 6 halves.

Calories: 34 *Fat: 1.5 grams*
Protein: 5 grams *Fibre: 0 gram*
Carbohydrates: 1 gram
Sodium: 130 milligrams

SHAKES

Basic Protein Shake and Deluxe (Chocolate or Vanilla)

Basic Protein Shake

4–6 fl. ounces non-fat milk
5 tablespoons protein powder (chocolate or vanilla)
Ice

Blend until smooth. Makes 1 serving.

Calories: 178 *Fat: 0.3 gram*
Protein: 26 grams *Fibre: 1 gram*
Carbohydrates: 13 grams
Sodium: 154 milligrams

Basic Protein Shake Deluxe

12–16 fl. ounces non-fat milk
10 tablespoons protein powder (chocolate or vanilla)
Ice

Blend until smooth. Makes 1 serving.

Calories: 356 *Fat: 0.6 gram*
Protein: 52 grams *Fibre: 2 grams*
Carbohydrates: 26 grams
Sodium: 300 milligrams

Banana Cream Shake and Deluxe

Banana Cream Shake

Follow directions for Basic Protein Shake (page 169), using vanilla protein powder and adding 1 small banana. Makes 1 serving.

Calories: 271 *Fat: 1 gram*
Protein: 27 grams *Fibre: 3 grams*
Carbohydrates: 37 grams
Sodium: 155 milligrams

Banana Cream Shake Deluxe

Follow directions for Basic Protein Shake Deluxe (page 169), using vanilla protein powder and adding 1 small banana. Makes 1 serving.

Calories: 449 *Fat: 1.3 grams*
Protein: 53 grams *Fibre: 4.4 grams*
Carbohydrates: 49 grams
Sodium: 310 milligrams

Strawberry Shake and Deluxe

Strawberry Shake

Follow directions for Basic Protein Shake (page 169), using vanilla protein powder and adding 5 ounces fresh or frozen strawberries. Makes 1 serving.

Calories: 223 *Fat: 0.9 gram*
Protein: 27 grams *Fibre: 4.5 grams*
Carbohydrates: 24 grams
Sodium: 156 milligrams

Strawberry Shake Deluxe

Follow directions for Basic Protein Shake Deluxe (page 169), using vanilla protein powder and adding 7½ ounces fresh or frozen strawberries. Makes 1 serving.

Calories: 425 *Fat: 1.5 grams*
Protein: 54 grams *Fibre: 7 grams*
Carbohydrates: 42 grams
Sodium: 310 milligrams

Strawberry–Banana Shake and Deluxe

Strawberry–Banana Shake

Follow directions for Basic Protein Shake (page 169), using vanilla protein powder. Add 5 ounces fresh or frozen strawberries and 1 small banana. Makes 1 serving.

Calories: 317 *Fat: 1 grams*
Protein: 28 grams *Fibre: 7 grams*
Carbohydrates: 47 grams
Sodium: 157 milligrams

Strawberry–Banana Shake Deluxe

Follow directions for Basic Protein Shake Deluxe (page 169), using vanilla protein powder. Add 7½ cups fresh or frozen strawberries and 1 small banana. Makes 1 serving.

Calories: 495 *Fat: 1.9 grams*
Protein: 54 grams *Fibre: 8 grams*
Carbohydrates: 60 grams
Sodium: 311 milligrams

French Vanilla Shake and Deluxe

French Vanilla Shake

Follow directions for Basic Protein Shake (page 169), using vanilla protein powder. Add 1 tablespoon fat-free French vanilla coffee creamer. Makes 1 serving.

Calories: 208 *Fat: 0.3 gram*
Protein: 26 grams *Fibre: 1 gram*
Carbohydrates: 20 grams
Sodium: 159 milligrams

French Vanilla Shake Deluxe

Follow directions for Basic Protein Shake Deluxe (page 169), using vanilla protein powder. Add 2 tablespoons fat-free French vanilla coffee creamer. Makes 1 serving.

Calories: 416 *Fat: 0.6 gram*
Protein: 52 grams *Fibre: 2 grams*
Carbohydrates: 40 grams
Sodium: 310 milligrams

Peanut Butter Shake and Deluxe

Peanut Butter Shake

Follow directions for Protein Shake (page 169), using vanilla or chocolate protein powder. Add 1 tablespoon peanut butter. Makes 1 serving.

Calories: 273 *Fat: 8.5 grams*
Protein: 30 grams *Fibre: 2 grams*
Carbohydrates: 16 grams
Sodium: 229 milligrams

Peanut Butter Shake Deluxe

Follow directions for Protein Shake Deluxe (page 169), using vanilla or chocolate protein powder. Add 2 tablespoons peanut butter. Makes 1 serving.

Calories: 546 *Fat: 17 grams*
Protein: 60 grams *Fibre: 4 grams*
Carbohydrates: 32 grams
Sodium: 458 milligrams

Peanut Butter–Strawberry Shake and Deluxe

Peanut Butter–Strawberry Shake

Follow directions for Basic Protein Shake (page 169), using vanilla or chocolate protein powder. Add 1 tablespoon peanut butter and 5 ounces cup fresh or frozen strawberries. Makes 1 serving.

Calories: 319 *Fat: 9 grams*
Protein: 31 grams *Fibre: 5 grams*
Carbohydrates: 27 grams
Sodium: 230 milligrams

Peanut Butter–Strawberry Shake Deluxe

Follow directions for Basic Protein Shake Deluxe (page 169), using vanilla or chocolate protein powder. Add 2 tablespoons peanut butter and 7½ ounces fresh or frozen strawberries. Makes 1 serving.

Calories: 592 *Fat: 18 grams*
Protein: 61 grams *Fibre: 7 grams*
Carbohydrates: 43 grams
Sodium: 459 milligrams

Cappuccino Shake

3 ounces cold brewed coffee
3 ounces non-fat milk
5 tablespoons vanilla protein powder
Ice

Blend ingredients until smooth. Makes 1 serving.

Calories: 145 *Fat: 2 grams*
Protein: 25 grams *Fibre: 1 gram*
Carboydrates: 9 grams
Sodium: 105 milligrams

Mocha Shake and Deluxe

Mocha Shake

4 ounces cold brewed coffee
5 tablespoons chocolate protein powder
Ice

Blend ingredients until smooth. Makes 1 serving.

Calories: 115 *Fat: 2 grams*
Protein: 20 grams *Fibre: 1 gram*
Carbohydrates: 4 grams
Sodium: 60 milligrams

Deluxe Mocha Shake

8 ounces cold brewed coffee
10 tablespoons chocolate protein powder
Ice

Blend ingredients until smooth. Makes 1 serving.

Calories: 230 *Fat: 4 grams*
Protein: 40 grams *Fibre: 2 grams*
Carbohydrates: 8 grams
Sodium: 120 milligrams

Washington Apple Salsa Chicken

by Sandi Anderson

Salsa

8 ounces chopped apple (Gala or Fuji)
3 ounces seeded and chopped Anaheim chilli peppers
2 ounces chopped onion
2 fl. ounces lime juice
2 tablespoons chopped cilantro

Marinade

2 fl. ounces white wine
2 fl. ounces apple juice
½ teaspoon grated lime zest

Chicken

2½ pounds boneless, skinless chicken breast

Mix salsa and let stand for at least 30 minutes.

Make marinade and marinate chicken for at least 20 minutes. After chicken marinates, bake it in the oven at 350°F/180°C/GM4 for 45 minutes or grill it on a barbecue on low heat for 16 to 20 minutes, turning after 8 minutes, until middle is not pink or thermometer reads 170°F/150°C. Serve salsa over cooked chicken. Makes 6 servings.

Calories: 365 *Fat: 6 grams*
Protein: 58 grams *Fibre: 0 gram*
Carbohydrates: 10 grams
Sodium: 144 milligrams

BBQ Chicken Breast

Quick and Large-Volume Recipe

2 pounds boneless, skinless chicken breast
8 tablespoons barbecue sauce (hickory or original)

Heat gas barbecue on high for 5 minutes. Reduce heat to low and spray grill with non-stick cooking spray. Place chicken breasts on grill and cook for 8 minutes. Turn chicken over and coat the cooked side of chicken with 1 tablespoon barbecue sauce. Cook chicken for another 8 minutes until middle is not pink or thermometer reads 170°F/150°C. Makes eight 4-ounce servings.

Calories: 146 *Fat: 3 grams*
Protein: 26 grams *Fibre: 0 gram*
Carbohydrates: 1 gram
Sodium: 324 milligrams

Oven-Fried Chicken

Quick and Large-Volume Recipe

8 ounces cornflakes crushed
1 tablespoon garlic powder
1 teaspoon seasoning salt
1 teaspoon paprika
4 pounds boneless, skinless chicken breast
16 fl. ounces skimmed milk

Preheat oven to 400°F/200°C/GM6. Line baking pan with foil. Mix dry ingredients in a quart-sized plastic bag. Dip chicken in milk, then place in bag and shake until chicken is coated. Place on prepared pan. Cook chicken for 20 to 25 minutes until middle is not pink or thermometer reads 170°F/150°C. Makes 20 3-ounce servings.

Calories: 161 *Fat: 3 grams*
Protein: 28 grams *Fibre: 0 gram*
Carbohydrates: 3 grams
Sodium: 408 milligrams

Sizzlin' Grilled Chicken Breast

Sizzlin' Grilling Marinade (page 184)
2 pounds boneless, skinless chicken breast

Make marinade. Marinate chicken breast for at least 2 hours. Heat gas barbecue on high for 5 minutes. Reduce heat to low and spray grill with non-stick cooking spray. Cook chicken breast for 8 to 10 minutes on each side until middle is no longer pink or thermometer reads 170°F/150°C. Makes eight 4-ounce servings.

Calories: 143 *Fat: 3 grams*
Protein: 26 grams *Fibre: 0 gram*
Carbohydrates: 1 gram
Sodium: 260 milligrams

Baked Soy Sauce Chicken

Large-Volume Recipe

5 pounds skinless, boneless chicken breast
4 fl. ounces reduced-sodium soy sauce
2 tablespoons garlic powder
Water

Preheat oven to 350°F/180°C/GM4. Place chicken in glass baking dish. Pour soy sauce over chicken. Sprinkle with garlic powder. Add enough water to fill dish with one inch of liquid. Cover with foil and bake for 1 hour until middle is not pink or thermometer reads 170°F/150°C. Makes 12 6-ounce servings.

Calories: 284 *Fat: 6 grams*
Protein: 53 grams *Fibre: 0 gram*
Carbohydrates: 0 gram
Sodium: 300 milligrams

Apple–Turkey Kabobs

8 fl. ounces apple juice
2 tablespoons Worcestershire sauce
½ teaspoon lemon pepper
1 tablespoon garlic powder
1½ pounds boneless, skinless turkey breast, cut into 1-inch cubes
Apple BBQ Sauce (page 185)
2 medium apples cut into wedges
1 large green pepper cut into wedges
18 mushrooms

Combine apple juice, Worcestershire sauce, lemon pepper, and garlic powder in a large resealable plastic bag; add turkey breast cubes. Seal bag; turn to coat. Marinate in refrigerator for 2 hours. Heat gas barbecue grill on high, then turn to low heat for cooking. Prepare Apple BBQ Sauce; set it aside. Remove turkey from marinade and alternately thread turkey, apple, and vegetables onto skewers. Spray grill with nonstick cooking spray. Place kabobs on grill. Grill for 10 to 12 minutes, turning after 6 minutes, and occasionally brushing with Apple BBQ Sauce until turkey is not pink and juice is clear. Makes 6 servings.

Calories: 173 *Fat: 1 gram*
Protein: 29 grams *Fibre: 2 grams*
Carbohydrates: 11 grams
Sodium: 142 milligrams

Chicken Brochettes

by Rosalie McPherson

1 pound skinless, boneless chicken breast
24 button mushrooms (two 8-ounce packages)
1½ tablespoons *herbes de Provence* or Italian seasoning
2½ tablespoons lime juice
1½ tablespoons honey
1 teaspoon salt
½ teaspoon black pepper
12 8-inch skewers

Cut chicken breast into 24 pieces. Remove stems from mushrooms. Cook *herbes de Provence* in a small frying pan with non-stick cooking spray over medium-low heat for 1 minute. Remove from heat and let cool. Stir in lime juice, honey, salt, and pepper. Place mushrooms and half of herb mixture in a large resealable plastic bag. Place chicken and remaining herb mixture in another resealable bag. Seal bags and marinate in the refrigerator for 1 hour, turning bags occasionally. Remove chicken and mushrooms from the bags and discard marinade. Preheat gas barbecue on high for 5 minutes, then reduce to medium-low for cooking. Spray grill with non-stick cooking spray. Thread 4 mushrooms onto each of 6 skewers. Thread 4 chicken pieces onto each of the other 6 skewers. Place skewers on grill and cook over medium-low heat for 5 minutes or until chicken is no longer pink and juice is clear. Makes 6 servings (two skewers per serving).

Calories: 160 *Fat: 1 gram*
Protein: 25 grams *Fibre: 3 grams*
Carbohydrates: 8 grams
Sodium: 233 milligrams

Bistro Chicken

by Jan Lutz

6 boneless, skinless chicken breast halves
4 ounces chopped onion
2 garlic cloves, minced
2 ounces chopped celery
¼ ounce chopped fresh basil
½ ounce chopped fresh parsley
2 fl. ounces red wine vinegar
1½ ounces sliced black olives
½ ounce capers, drained
2 teaspoons sugar
Dash of ground red pepper
1 bay leaf
One 14½-ounce can Italian-style tomatoes, diced and drained

Spray a large frying pan with non-stick cooking spray and place over medium-high heat. Add chicken, and sauté on each side until lightly browned. Remove from pan. Spray pan again. Add onion and garlic and sauté until translucent. Add celery and sauté for 5 minutes. Add basil, parsley, vinegar, olives, capers, sugar, red pepper, bay leaf, and tomatoes. Return chicken to pan; bring to a boil. Cover, reduce heat, and simmer for 20 minutes. Serve over pasta or rice. Makes 6 servings (1 chicken breast half and 4 fl. ounces sauce per serving).

Calories: 208 *Fat: 3.6 grams*
Protein: 29 grams *Fibre: 2 grams*
Carbohydrates: 14 grams
Sodium: 490 milligrams

Turkey Salsa Burgers

Quick Recipe

2½ pounds ground turkey breast
6 ounces thick and chunky salsa
3 tablespoons garlic powder

Heat gas barbecue grill. Turn to low. Mix all ingredients in a large bowl. Form eight patties. Spray grill with non-stick cooking spray. Cook patties for 7 to 9 minutes on each side until turkey is white and thermometer reads 170°F/150°C. Do not overcook turkey or it will become very dry. Makes eight 3-ounce servings.

Calories: 133 | *Fat: 1.5 grams*
Protein: 27 grams | *Fibre: 0 gram*
Carbohydrates: 3 grams
Sodium: 230 milligrams

Turkey Meatloaf

Large-Volume Recipe

2 pounds ground turkey breast
2 tablespoons garlic powder
4 egg whites
3 slices non-fat cheese
4 fl. ounces barbecue sauce

Preheat oven to 350°F/180°C/GM4. Mix turkey breast, garlic powder, and egg whites together and place in rectangular 9×13 baking dish, forming a loaf. Cover with foil and bake for 45 minutes. Uncover and place cheese on top of loaf, then pour barbecue sauce over the top. Leave uncovered and bake for another 15 minutes until thermometer reads 170°F/150°C. Makes 8 servings.

Calories: 185 | *Fat: 2 grams*
Protein: 36 grams | *Fibre: 0.6 gram*
Carbohydrates: 7 grams
Sodium: 312 milligrams

Turkey Meatballs

by Rosalie McPherson

Quick and Large-Volume Recipe

2½ pounds ground turkey breast
1 ounce porridge oats, uncooked
9 ounces cooked brown rice
3 large egg whites
¼ teaspoon salt
1½ teaspoons dried, rubbed sage
¼ teaspoon dried thyme
1½ teaspoons onion powder
¼ teaspoon black pepper

Preheat oven to 425°F/220°C/GM7. Line a baking sheet with foil and spray foil with non-stick cooking spray. Mix all the ingredients together. Form 6 meatballs for every ¼ of mixture. Place on prepared pan. Bake for 4 to 6 minutes, then turn over and cook for another 4 to 6 minutes until centre of meatball has turned white. Makes about 24 meatballs.

Per meatball:
Calories: 91 *Fat: 0.5 gram*
Protein: 6 grams *Fibre: 1 gram*
Carbohydrates: 14 grams
Sodium: 172 milligrams

Grilled Pepper Steak

Quick

4 fl. ounces chicken broth
½ ounce chopped fresh parsley
1 ounce minced onion
2 tablespoons Worcestershire sauce
1 teaspoon freshly ground pepper
½ teaspoon dry mustard
2 pounds lean top sirloin steaks

Combine broth, parsley, onion, Worcestershire sauce, pepper, and mustard in a saucepan. Heat, stirring continually, for 3 minutes. Heat grill to medium-high and place steaks on grill rack. Brush frequently with pepper mixture. Depending on thickness of steaks, cook for 6 to 8 minutes on each side for medium. Makes 8 servings.

Calories: 175 *Fat: 7 grams*
Protein: 26 grams *Fibre: 0 gram*
Carbohydrates: 0 gram
Sodium: 89 milligrams

Marinated Flank Steak

by Jan Lutz

3 fl. ounces dry red wine
1 ounce chopped sweet onion
2 teaspoons reduced-sodium soy sauce
2 garlic cloves, minced
¼ teaspoon salt
¼ teaspoon pepper
1 pound lean flank steak

Combine wine, onion, soy sauce, garlic, salt, and pepper in a large resealable bag. Add steak to bag. Seal and marinate for at least 30 minutes, turning occasionally. Heat grill on high then turn to low and coat with non-stick cooking spray. Place steak on grill rack. Grill for 5 minutes on each side until desired degree of doneness. Cut steak diagonally across the grain in thin slices. Makes 4 servings.

Calories: 311 *Fat: 14 grams*
Protein: 36 grams *Fibre: 0 gram*
Carbohydrates: 1 gram
Sodium: 442 milligrams

Fish with Cucumber Relish

Quick

One 11-ounce can mandarin oranges, drained
1 small cucumber, peeled and finely chopped
3 fl. ounces rice vinegar
1 green onion, minced
1 tablespoon chopped fresh dill, plus sprigs for garnish
1 pound cod or orange roughy fillets

Reserve 8 mandarin orange sections for garnish. Coarsely chop remaining sections and combine with cucumber, vinegar, onion, and dill. Spray grill pan with non-stick cooking spray; place fish on pan. Spoon 1 tablespoon of cucumber mixture over each fillet. Broil for 8 to 10 minutes or until fish flakes easily with a fork. To serve, top with remaining relish mix and garnish with orange sections and dill sprigs. Makes 4 servings.

Calories: 146 *Fat: 1 gram*
Protein: 21 grams *Fibre: 1 gram*
Carbohydrates: 13 grams
Sodium: 67 milligrams

Microwaved Cod Fillets

Quick

1 pound cod or orange roughy fillets
6 ounces non-fat sour cream
6 ounces non-fat mayonnaise
3 tablespoons skimmed milk
1 tablespoon Dijon mustard
1½ teaspoons fresh dill

Cut fish into 4 pieces; place in a microwave-safe dish. Cover and microwave on high for 2 to 4 minutes. Drain and combine the sour cream, mayonnaise, milk, mustard, and dill. Drizzle half over fish and microwave uncovered for 3 to 4 minutes or until fish flakes easily with a fork. Makes 4 servings.

Calories: 128 *Fat: 1.3 grams*
Protein: 22 grams *Fibre: 0 gram*
Carbohydrates: 6 grams
Sodium: 164 milligrams

Grilled Salmon

4 fl. ounces reduced-sodium soy sauce
1 tablespoon brown sugar
2 fl. ounces lemon juice
1 teaspoon grated lemon peel
1 pound fresh salmon fillet

Mix first four ingredients in a large resealable plastic bag. Cut salmon into 4 pieces. Place salmon in bag and marinate for 1 hour. Preheat grill. Place fish in a pan sprayed with non-stick cooking spray. Broil on top rack for 3 to 4 minutes on each side until fish flakes easily with fork. Makes 4 4-ounce servings.

Calories: 342 *Fat: 19 grams*
Protein: 36 grams *Fibre: 0 gram*
Carbohydrates: 8 grams
Sodium: 1,061 milligrams

Foil-Baked Salmon

Quick

1 pound salmon
½ lemon, sliced thin
2 tablespoons lemon pepper

Preheat oven to 350°F/180°C/GM4. Place fish on a large piece of foil. Sprinkle lemon pepper over fish and lay lemon wedges on top of fish. Wrap fish in foil and bake for 20 minutes or until fish flakes with a fork. Makes 4 servings.

Calories: 326 *Fat: 18 grams*
Protein: 34 grams *Fibre: 0 gram*
Carbohydrates: 5 grams
Sodium: 101 milligrams

Sizzlin' Grilling Marinade

8 fl. ounces Worcestershire sauce
8 fl. ounces vinegar (red wine or rice)
4 fl. ounces teriyaki or gourmet sauce
1 tablespoon Dijon mustard
1 tablespoon garlic powder

Mix all ingredients together. Marinate steak, chicken, or turkey breasts for at least 2 hours. Cook meat over low heat on a grill to desired doneness. Makes 32 1-teaspoon servings.

Per teaspoon:
Calories: 9 *Fat: 0 gram*
Protein: 0 gram *Fibre: 0 gram*
Carbohydrates: 2 grams
Sodium: 205 milligrams

Spicy Marinade

2 fl. ounces reduced-sodium soy sauce
2 fl. ounces orange juice
2 teaspoons sugar substitute
2 garlic cloves, minced
1 teaspoon rum extract
¼ teaspoon ground ginger
1 teaspoon hot pepper sauce

Mix all ingredients together in a resealable plastic bag. Marinate uncooked chicken or turkey breast for 2 hours. Makes 4 fl. ounces.

Per teaspoon:
Calories: 21 *Fat: 0 gram*
Protein: 0 gram *Fibre: 0 gram*
Carbohydrates: 5 grams
Sodium: 301 milligrams

Apple BBQ Sauce

- 2 ounces chopped onion
- 4 fl. ounces apple juice
- 8 fl. ounces chilli sauce
- 6 ounces unsweetened applesauce
- 6 ounces sugar substitute
- 1 tablespoon Worcestershire sauce
- 1 teaspoon dry mustard
- 5 drops hot pepper sauce

Combine onion and apple juice in a 1-quart saucepan. Simmer for 2 minutes. Stir in chilli sauce, applesauce, sugar substitute, Worcestershire sauce, mustard, and hot pepper sauce. Simmer for 10 minutes. Makes 16 fl. ounces.

2 tablespoons:
Calories: 31 *Fat: 0 gram*
Protein: 0 gram *Fibre: 0 gram*
Carbohydrates: 8 grams
Sodium: 211 milligrams

MAIN ENTRÉES

Spaghetti Sauce

- 1 pound minced turkey breast
- 1 small onion, chopped
- 12 ounces sliced mushrooms
- 1 green pepper, diced
- 2 small courgettes, diced
- One 15-ounce can Italian stewed tomatoes
- Three 8-ounce cans tomato sauce
- 1 tablespoon garlic powder
- Two 6-ounce cans tomato paste
- 1 teaspoon *each* of dried oregano, dried basil, and salt (optional)

Spray an extra-large pan with non-stick cooking spray. Add meat and onion. Brown meat. Add the remaining ingredients. Simmer until vegetables are tender (1 to 2 hours). Makes 12 1-cup servings.

Per serving:
Calories: 101 *Fat: 0.6 gram*
Protein: 14 grams *Fibre: 3 grams*
Carbohydrates: 11 grams
Sodium: 467 milligrams

Vegetarian Spaghetti Sauce
Eliminate meat. This will decrease the calories to 61, protein to 6 grams, and fat to 0 gram.

Turkey Lasagne

1 pound minced turkey breast
1 tablespoon garlic powder
12 ounces mushrooms, sliced
1 green pepper, chopped
One 15-ounce can diced stewed tomatoes, drained
Two 8-ounce cans tomato sauce
Two 6-ounce cans tomato paste
1 teaspoon each of dried oregano, dried basil, and salt (optional)
10 wide lasagne noodles
16 ounces non-fat cottage cheese
4 egg whites
8 ounces non-fat shredded mozarella
8 ounces non-fat shredded Cheddar cheese

To make the meat sauce, brown meat with garlic powder in large pan coated with non-stick cooking spray. Add mushrooms, green pepper, stewed tomatoes, tomato sauce, tomato paste, and spices. Simmer for 30 minutes. Cook the noodles until tender. Mix cottage cheese and egg whites. Preheat oven to 350°F/180°C/GM4. Spray a 13×9 baking dish with non-stick cooking spray. Lay three noodles on the bottom of the pan. Spoon half of the meat sauce over the noodles. Spread on half of the cottage cheese mixture. Sprinkle on one-third of *each* cheese. Make another layer of noodles, then meat sauce, cottage cheese mixture, and cheeses. Place the last three noodles on the top. Sprinkle with the remaining cheeses. Cover with foil and bake for 1 hour. Cheese will be bubbly; insert knife in centre to make sure it is heated through. Makes 12 servings.

Calories: 219 *Fat: 1.5 grams*
Protein: 28 grams *Fibre: 2.6 grams*
Carbohydrates: 26 grams
Sodium: 702 milligram

Vegetarian Lasagne
Eliminate the turkey. This will reduce the calories to 175, protein to 17 grams, and fat to 1 gram.

Hearty Chilli

Large-Volume Recipe

1 pound minced turkey breast or 4% lean minced beef
1 small onion, diced
3 courgettes, sliced
1 green pepper, chopped
1 large carrot, chopped
One 15-ounce can stewed tomatoes
Three 15-ounce cans low-sodium kidney beans
One 15-ounce can black beans
Three 15-ounce cans tomato sauce
2 teaspoons chilli powder
1 tablespoon garlic powder
1 teaspoon salt (optional)
Two 8-ounce cans tomato paste

Vegetarian Chilli
Eliminate the meat. This will reduce the calories to 169, protein to 14 grams, and fat to 0.2 gram.

Brown meat in a large stock pot or electric slow cooker. Add the remaining ingredients and cover. Simmer over low heat, stirring occasionally, until vegetables are tender, 1 to 3 hours. Makes 20 1-cup servings.

Calories: 197 *Fat: 1 gram*
Protein: 20 grams *Fibre: 8 grams*
Carbohydrates: 28 grams
Sodium: 814 milligrams

Beef Stew

Large-Volume Recipe

2 pounds flank steak
1 small onion
Two 15-ounce cans tomato sauce
12 ounces mushrooms, sliced
1 pound baby carrots, cut into chunks
1 pound red potatoes with skin, cut into chunks
2 tablespoons garlic powder
4 courgettes, cut into 1-inch chunks
1 teaspoon dried basil
1 teaspoon salt (optional)
5 pints water
12 chicken stock cubes

Cut meat into 1-inch cubes. In large stock pot, brown meat with onions. Add tomato sauce and cook over low heat for 30 minutes. Add the remaining ingredients. Simmer for 1 to 3 hours until potatoes are tender. Makes 16 servings.

Calories: 192 *Fat: 3 grams*
Protein: 19 grams *Fibre: 2 grams*
Carbohydrates: 19 grams
Sodium: 396 milligrams

Oriental Chicken Noodle Soup

3 pints water
8 stock cubes
7 ounces whole-wheat spaghetti
1 celery stalk, chopped
1 large carrot, chopped
1 tablespoon reduced-sodium soy sauce
12½ ounces canned chicken breast

Heat water in a large saucepan over high heat and dissolve bouillon cubes. Add spaghetti, celery, carrot, and soy sauce. Cook until tender. Add chicken and simmer over low heat for 15 minutes. Makes 8 servings.

Calories: 171 *Fat: 2 grams*
Protein: 18 grams *Fibre: 0 gram*
Carbohydrates: 20 grams
Sodium: 1,001 milligrams

Angel Hair Pasta with Chicken

12 ounces boneless, skinless chicken breast, cubed
1 large carrot, sliced diagonally into ¼-inch pieces
6 ounces chicken broth, divided
2 garlic cloves, minced
One 10-ounce package frozen broccoli florets
12 ounces angel hair pasta
1 teaspoon dried basil
½ ounce grated Parmesan cheese

Spray medium pan with non-stick cooking spray. Heat over medium-high heat and add chicken. Cook, stirring, until chicken is cooked through, about 5 minutes. Remove from pan. In a separate pot, begin heating water for pasta. In pan, add carrot and 3 tablespoons of the chicken broth and cook for 4 minutes. Add garlic and broccoli to pan and cook for another 2 minutes. Cook pasta according to directions. While pasta is cooking, add rest of chicken broth, basil, and chicken to pan. Simmer for 4 minutes. Drain pasta and place in a large serving bowl. Top with chicken mixture and then cheese. Makes 4 servings.

Calories: 493 *Fat: 6.5 grams*
Protein: 44 grams *Fibre: 2 grams*
Carbohydrates: 68 grams
Sodium: 534 milligrams

Chicken or Shrimp Jambalaya

by Jan Lutz

1 medium onion, chopped
2 garlic cloves, minced
1 pound chicken breast cut into ¾-inch pieces or 1 pound shrimp, deveined
One 14½-ounce can whole plum tomatoes
1 tablespoon tomato paste
1 celery stalk, cut into ½-inch slices
1 small green pepper, chopped
1 whole spring onion
1 bay leaf
1 teaspoon dried thyme
Pinch ground cloves
¼ teaspoon red pepper flakes
4 ounces lean ham, cut into ½-inch cubes
6 ounces cooked long-grain brown rice

In a large pot, sauté onion and garlic in non-stick cooking spray over medium-high heat for about 4 minutes. Add chicken and cook, stirring, until the pieces are white on all sides. Add undrained tomatoes and the remaining ingredients *except* ham and rice. Bring to boil and simmer until chicken is cooked and sauce has thickened, about 20 minutes. Mix ham and rice into the chicken mixture, heat, and serve. Makes 6 servings.

Calories: 169 *Fat: 2 grams*
Protein: 23 grams *Fibre: 2 grams*
Carbohydrates: 14 grams
Sodium: 439 milligrams

Turkey Rice Mix

by Blair McHaney

Large-Volume Recipe

18 ounces brown rice
$3\frac{1}{3}$ pounds ground turkey breast
***Optional seasonings:* garlic, Italian, taco, pepper, salsa, or seasoned rice vinegar**
***Optional:* 9 ounces mixed vegetables (broccoli, green beans, stir-fry vegetable mixture) or 12 ounces chopped apples**

Cook the rice. Cook the turkey breast with the seasoning of your choice. Mix the rice and turkey in a very large bowl. Using quart-size containers or plastic bags for refrigeration or freezing, fill each bag or container evenly until mixture is gone. Decide how many bags you will need from the breakdown below. (Adding vegetables or apples will add a small amount of calories. This will also add extra fibre and variety.) This recipe is also tasty when the seasoning is not added until the dish is reheated. Use these prepared meals for between-meal snacks or main entrées. Makes 10, 12, or 15 servings.

Servings	**Calories**	**Protein (grams)**	**Fat (grams)**	**Carbs (grams)**	**Fibre (grams)**	**Sodium (mg)**
10	387	39	2.6	47	3	137
12	322	32	2.2	39.5	2.5	119
15	258	26	1.75	31.5	2	106

Chicken Stir-Fry

1 pound boneless, skinless chicken breast
1 small onion, chopped
1 green or red pepper, sliced
12 ounces broccoli flowerets
12 ounces mushrooms, sliced
12 ounces sugar snap peas
6 ounces bean sprouts

Cut chicken into strips. Heat wok or large pan coated with non-stick cooking spray over high heat. Brown chicken. Add onion and green pepper. Sauté on medium heat for 3 minutes. Add remaining ingredients, cover, and cook until crisp-tender, 5 to 6 minutes. Makes 4 servings.

Calories: 319 *Fat: 5 grams*
Protein: 43 grams *Fibre: 12 grams*
Carbohydrates: 30 grams
Sodium: 212 milligrams

Tasty Brown Rice

Brown, basmati, wild, or long-grain rice
Stock cubes or fat-free chicken broth
Water

Prepare rice as directed on package. For each cup of water, use one stock cube or replace water with fat-free chicken broth only. Cook as directed.

1-cup serving:
Calories: 235 *Fat: 1 gram*
Protein: 5 grams *Fibre: 3 grams*
Carbohydrates: 50 grams
Sodium: 1,126 milligrams

Chicken Apple Stir-Fry

by Royce Tigner

4 ounces dried mushrooms, shiitake or wood ear
12 ounces skinless, boneless chicken breast
6 fl. ounces cold water
3 tablespoons frozen orange juice concentrate, thawed
2 tablespoons low-sodium soy sauce
2 teaspoons cornstarch
¼ teaspoon ground ginger
¼ teaspoon ground cinnamon
¼ teaspoon ground red pepper
3 tablespoons sliced or slivered almonds
2 medium green peppers, cut into 2-inch strips
2 medium apples, thinly sliced

In a small bowl, add warm water to mushrooms to cover and soak for 30 minutes. Rinse and squeeze mushrooms to drain thoroughly. Discard stems. Thinly slice mushrooms and set aside. Cut chicken into 1-inch pieces. Set aside. In a small bowl, stir together water, orange juice concentrate, soy sauce, cornstarch, ginger, cinnamon, and red pepper. Set aside. Preheat pan or wok over medium-high heat. Spray with non-stick cooking spray and add almonds; stir-fry for 2 to 3 minutes or until golden. Remove almonds from pan. Spray pan with non-stick cooking spray. Add mushrooms, green peppers, and apples; stir-fry for 1 to 2 minutes or until peppers and apples are crisp-tender. Remove apple mixture from pan. Add chicken to pan and stir-fry for 3 to 4 minutes or until browned. Push chicken away from the centre of the pan. Stir orange juice mixture and add to the centre of the pan. Cook and stir until sauce is thickened and bubbly. Return apple mixture to the wok. Stir all ingredients together to coat with sauce. Cook and stir for 1 to 2 minutes or until heated thoroughly. Stir in toasted almonds. Makes 4 servings.

Calories: 220 *Fat: 5 grams*
Protein: 24 grams *Fibre: 4.5 grams*
Carbohydrates: 22 grams
Sodium: 180 milligrams
Served over 3 ounces brown rice:
Calories: 337 *Fat: 5 grams*
Protein: 26 grams *Fibre: 6 grams*
Carbohydrates: 47 grams
Sodium: 195 milligrams

Beef or Chicken Fajitas

1 small onion, cut in strips
1 green pepper, cut in strips
1 red pepper, cut in strips
Fat-free chicken broth
1 pound cooked top-sirloin or chicken breast strips
1 tablespoon chilli powder
1 tablespoon garlic powder
5 whole-wheat tortillas

With 3 ounces of chicken breast:
Calories: 236 *Fat: 3.5 grams*
Protein: 30 grams *Fibre: 2.6 grams*
Carbohydrates: 26 grams
Sodium: 494 milligrams

In a pan, sauté onions and peppers in broth over medium heat until tender. In same pan, add meat to one side of the pan. Add chilli and garlic powders and simmer for 20 minutes on low heat. Heat tortillas in microwave. On each tortilla, place ⅕ (3 ounces) meat and one-fifth onion-pepper mixture and roll up. Makes 5 tortillas.

With 3 ounces of beef:
Calories: 260 *Fat: 6 grams*
Protein: 29 grams *Fibre: 2.6 grams*
Carbohydrates: 26 grams
Sodium: 495 milligrams

Whole-Wheat Tortilla Tacos

1 pound minced turkey breast or 4% lean minced beef
1 packet taco seasoning mix
5 whole-wheat tortillas
5 ounces non-fat shredded Cheddar cheese
Lettuce
Salsa

With 3 ounces of beef and one tablespoon salsa:
Calories: 278 *Fat: 7 grams*
Protein: 35 grams *Fibre: 2 grams*
Carbohydrates: 22 grams
Sodium: 969 milligrams

Spray a pan with non-stick cooking spray and cook meat over medium heat until browned. Follow the directions for using the seasoning mix. Warm tortillas in microwave for 10 to 15 seconds. Put about 3 ounces meat and 1 ounce cheese on each tortilla and roll up. Add desired amount of lettuce and salsa. Makes 5 servings.

With 3 ounces of turkey breast and one tablespoon salsa:
Calories: 207 *Fat: 2 grams*
Protein: 32 grams *Fibre: 2 grams*
Carbohydrates: 23 grams
Sodium: 981 milligrams

Corn Tortilla Tacos

1 pound minced turkey breast or 4% lean minced beef
1 packet taco seasoning mix
Ten 4-inch corn tortillas
5 ounces non-fat shredded Cheddar cheese
Lettuce
Salsa

Spray a pan with non-stick cooking spray and cook meat over medium heat until browned. Follow the directions for using the seasoning mix. Warm corn tortillas in microwave for 10 to 15 seconds. Put about 1½ ounces meat and ½ ounce cheese on each tortilla and roll up. Add desired amount of lettuce and salsa. Makes 10 tortillas or 5 servings.

With 3 ounces beef and one tablespoon salsa:
Calories: 240 *Fat: 7 grams*
Protein: 33 grams *Fibre: 1 gram*
Carbohydrates: 10 grams
Sodium: 812 milligrams

With 3 ounces turkey breast and one tablespoon salsa:
Calories: 170 *Fat: 2 grams*
Protein: 30 grams *Fibre: 1 gram*
Carbohydrates: 10 grams
Sodium: 825 milligrams

Bean Burrito

14 ounces non-fat refried beans
4 ounces of non-fat shredded Cheddar cheese
8 tablespoons salsa
4 whole-wheat tortillas

Place ¼ of the beans, 1 ounce cheese, and 2 tablespoons salsa on each tortilla. Roll up and place all tortillas seamside down in a microwave-safe baking dish. Heat for 2 to 3 minutes until cheese melts. Makes 4 servings.

Calories: 213 *Fat: 1 gram*
Protein: 15 grams *Fibre: 6.5 grams*
Carbohydrates: 42 grams
Sodium: 644 milligrams

Beef Burrito

1 pound 4% minced beef
5 whole-wheat tortillas
5 ounces non-fat shredded Cheddar cheese
Salsa
Garlic powder or other seasoning

Spray pan with non-stick cooking spray and brown meat with seasoning over medium heat and drain. Heat tortillas in microwave for 10 to 15 seconds. Place about 3 ounces meat, 1 ounce cheese, and desired amount salsa on each tortilla and roll up. Heat seamside down on plate in microwave for 25 seconds. Makes 5 servings.

Calories: 277 *Fat: 7 grams*
Protein: 35 grams *Fibre: 2 grams*
Carbohydrates: 22 grams
Sodium: 487 milligrams

Beef and Bean Burrito

1 pound 4% minced beef
Garlic powder or other seasoning
5 whole-wheat tortillas
5 ounces non-fat shredded Cheddar cheese
9 ounces non-fat refried beans
Salsa

Spray pan with non-stick cooking spray and brown meat and seasoning over medium heat and drain. Heat tortillas in microwave for 10 to 15 seconds. Place about 3 ounces meat, 1 ounce cheese, ⅕ of the beans, and desired amount salsa on each tortilla and roll up. Heat seamside down on plate in microwave for 2 to 3 minutes until cheese melts. Makes 5 servings.

Calories: 331 *Fat: 7 grams*
Protein: 38 grams *Fibre: 4 grams*
Carbohydrates: 32 grams
Sodium: 587 milligrams

"No Stick 'um" Apple Pizza

by Mary Ellen Kerby

Crust

7½ ounces stone-ground whole-wheat flour
1 tablespoon sugar substitute
1 package yeast (dissolved in 4 fl. ounces hot water)
½ teaspoon salt
1 tablespoon unsweetened applesauce
1 tablespoon olive oil
½ teaspoon vanilla flavouring

Topping

¾ tablespoon light margarine
Cinnamon and sugar substitute
8 ounces shredded low-fat mozzarella or Cheddar cheese
4 medium apples, peeled and thinly sliced

To make the crust, mix the dry ingredients in a bowl, then add liquids. Roll out the crust and place it on a 12-inch pizza pan. Preheat oven to 375°F/190°C/GM5. Brush the dough with margarine. Sprinkle cinnamon and sugar substitute evenly over the dough. Spread cheese over the dough, and place apple slices on top of cheese. Sprinkle again with cinnamon and sugar substitute. Bake for 25 minutes. Makes 8 servings.

Calories: 181 *Fat: 3 grams*
Protein: 9.6 grams *Fibre: 4.6 grams*
Carbohydrates: 31 grams
Sodium: 596 milligrams

Sweet Tater Surprise

by Nancy Van Hoven

1 medium sweet potato, cooked
3 fl. ounces water
1 ounce porridge oats, uncooked
3 tablespoons vanilla protein powder

Remove skin from cooked sweet potato and discard. Mash the pulp. Mix with water, oatmeal, and protein powder.

Calories: 238 *Fat: 0.8 gram*
Protein: 11 grams *Fibre: 7 grams*
Carbohydrates: 48 grams
Sodium: 29 milligrams

Waldorf Salad

3 ounces cooked chicken breast
4 ounces spinach, chopped
1 medium apple, chopped
½ tablespoon walnuts
1 teaspoon raisins
2 tablespoons non-fat salad dressing (honey mustard or Catalina)

Dice chicken breast. Toss all ingredients together and add salad dressing. Makes 1 serving.

Calories: 313 *Fat: 6 grams*
Protein: 29 grams *Fibre: 7 grams*
Carbohydrates: 38 grams
Sodium: 398 milligrams

Grilled Chicken Caesar Salad

3 ounces grilled chicken breast
6 ounces romaine lettuce, chopped
1 tablespoon shredded Parmesan cheese
2 tablespoons non-fat Caesar salad dressing

Cut chicken breast into strips. Mix all ingredients in a bowl and serve. Makes 1 serving.

Calories: 192 *Fat: 5 grams*
Protein: 30 grams *Fibre: 2 grams*
Carbohydrates: 6 grams
Sodium: 345 milligrams

Chicken–Broccoli Salad

3 ounces canned chicken breast
3 ounces broccoli, chopped
6 ounces romaine lettuce, chopped
2 tablespoons non-fat salad dressing
½ tablespoon shredded Parmesan cheese

Cut chicken into 1-inch cubes. Toss with lettuce, broccoli, and salad dressing. Sprinkle with parmesan. Makes 1 serving.

Calories: 221 *Fat: 4 grams*
Protein: 31 grams *Fibre: 5 grams*
Carbohydrates: 16 grams
Sodium: 602 milligrams

Chicken–Apple Salad

14 ounces diced red apples
2 tablespoons lemon juice
2 ounces non-fat mayonnaise
2 tablespoons non-fat sour cream
12 ounces grapes
1 celery stalk, diced
1 large carrot, shredded
9 ounces romaine lettuce, chopped
12 ounces canned chicken breast
1½ ounces walnut pieces

Mix apples with lemon juice. In separate bowl, mix mayonnaise and sour cream. Add remaining ingredients to the apples. Toss; add mayonnaise mixture and mix well. Makes 8 servings.

Calories: 200 *Fat: 4 grams*
Protein: 11 grams *Fibre: 4 grams*
Carbohydrates: 33 grams
Sodium: 935 milligrams

Smoked Turkey–Apple Salad

by Gloria and Stanley Arbogast

Dressing

1 tablespoon olive oil
1 tablespoon Dijon mustard
2 tablespoons apple cider vinegar
1 teaspoon lemon pepper

Salad

1 carrot, julienned
10 cherry tomatoes, halved
8 ounces smoked turkey breast, julienned
4 unpeeled apples, diced
1½ pounds romaine lettuce, chopped
2 tablespoons chopped walnuts, toasted

Make dressing. Set aside. Mix carrot, tomatoes, turkey, and apples. Arrange lettuce on a platter or plates. Top with salad ingredients, drizzle salad dressing on top, and sprinkle with walnuts. Makes 4 servings.

Calories: 209 *Fat: 7 grams*
Protein: 15 grams *Fibre: 4.5 grams*
Carbohydrates: 24 grams
Sodium: 817 milligrams

Oriental Salmon Salad

- 4½ ounces shredded red cabbage
- 1½ pounds shredded Chinese cabbage
- 10 ounces shredded carrots
- 4 ounces sliced spring onions
- One 10-ounce can mandarin oranges
- 1 ounce slivered almonds
- One 16-ounce bottle non-fat Oriental dressing
- 6 ounces salmon
- 5 ounces rice noodles

Mix all ingredients together *except* salmon and noodles. Gently mix in salmon and top with rice noodles. Makes 6 servings.

Calories: 363 *Fat: 5.8 grams*
Protein: 12 grams *Fibre: 4 grams*
Carbohydrates: 65 grams
Sodium: 723 milligrams

Steak Salad

- ½ green pepper, cut into strips
- ½ small onion, cut in strips
- 3 ounces grilled top-sirloin steak
- 6 ounces chopped romaine lettuce
- 4 ounces spinach
- 2 tablespoons non-fat ranch dressing

Sauté pepper and onion in a pan with non-stick cooking spray over medium-high heat until crisp-tender. Cut steak into strips and add to pan. Heat for 2 minutes. Combine lettuce and spinach and put in a salad bowl. Add dressing and toss until evenly distributed. Add meat mixture and serve. Makes 1 serving.

Calories: 237 *Fat: 6 grams*
Protein: 29 grams *Fibre: 5 grams*
Carbohydrates: 17 grams
Sodium: 362 milligrams

Tuna–Mixed Green Salad

6 ounces chopped romaine lettuce
4 ounces chopped spinach
1 small tomato, diced
6 ounces tuna in water, drained
2 tablespoons non-fat Italian dressing

Combine lettuce, spinach, and tomato and put in a salad bowl. Toss in tuna and mix. Add dressing. Makes 1 serving.

Calories: 268 *Fat: 2 grams*
Protein: 46 grams *Fibre: 3 grams*
Carbohydrates: 14 grams
Sodium: 961 milligrams

Taco Salad

1 pound 4% lean minced beef or minced turkey breast
1 packet taco seasoning mix
1½ pounds chopped mixed green lettuce
4 ounces non-fat Cheddar cheese
16 fl. ounces salsa

Cook meat until brown. Add taco seasoning to meat as directed on package. Divide lettuce among 4 bowls. Add one-quarter meat, 1 ounce cheese, and 4 fl. ounces salsa over lettuce in each bowl. Makes 4 servings.

Calories: 236 *Fat: 5 grams*
Protein: 30 grams *Fibre: 7 grams*
Carbohydrates: 19 grams
Sodium: 1,137 milligrams

Grilled Salmon Salad

3 ounces grilled salmon
6 ounces chopped romaine lettuce
4 ounces chopped courgettes
1 medium apple, chopped
2 tablespoon seasoned rice vinegar

Mix lettuce with remaining ingredients in a salad bowl. Makes 1 serving.

Calories: 288 *Fat: 7 grams*
Protein: 22 grams *Fibre: 11 grams*
Carbohydrates: 27 grams
Sodium: 64 milligrams

Salmon Caesar Salad

3 ounces salmon, canned or grilled
6 ounces chopped romaine lettuce
1 tablespoon shredded Parmesan cheese
2 tablespoons non-fat Caesar salad dressing

Break salmon into chunks. Mix with remaining ingredients. Makes 1 serving.

Calories: 174 *Fat: 7.5 grams*
Protein: 21 grams *Fibre: 2 grams*
Carbohydrates: 6 grams
Sodium: 438 milligrams

Fresh Vegetable Stir-Fry

1 tablespoon cornstarch
½ teaspoon salt
8 fl. ounces fat-free chicken broth
¼ pound French beans, cut into 1½-inch pieces
3 small onions, chopped
1 large garlic clove, minced
1 medium courgette, chopped
1 large green or red pepper, cut into thin strips
2½ ounces thinly sliced carrots
1 medium tomato, cut into wedges
¼ ounce minced fresh basil
1 teaspoon lemon juice (optional)

In a small bowl, stir cornstarch, salt, and broth until smooth; set aside. Spray large pan with non-stick cooking spray and heat over medium-high heat. Add beans, onions, and garlic; cook, stirring quickly and frequently, for 2 minutes. Add courgette, pepper, and carrots; stir-fry for 2 to 3 minutes or until all vegetables are crisp-tender. Stir cornstarch mixture and add to pan. Stir constantly and bring to a boil over medium heat for 1 minute. Stir in tomato, basil, and lemon juice; cook for another minute. Makes 6 servings.

Calories: 73 *Fat: 0.5 gram*
Protein: 4 grams *Fibre: 6 grams*
Carbohydrates: 6 grams
Sodium: 183 milligrams

Asparagus Stir-Fry

1 tablespoon cornstarch
6 fl. ounces reduced-sodium chicken broth plus 1 tablespoon
2 tablespoons reduced-sodium soy sauce
¾ pound fresh asparagus, trimmed and cut into 2-inch pieces
½ medium green pepper, julienned
1 ounce sliced spring onions
1 garlic clove, minced
8 ounces sliced mushrooms
One 8-ounce can water chestnuts, drained

In a small bowl, combine cornstarch, broth, and soy sauce until smooth; set aside. In a large pan or wok, stir-fry asparagus, green pepper, onions, and garlic in 1 tablespoon of hot chicken broth for 2 to 3 minutes. Add mushrooms; stir-fry for 1 to 2 minutes. Add water chestnuts; stir-fry for 1 to 2 minutes longer. Stir cornstarch mixture; add to vegetables. Bring to boil; cook and stir for 2 minutes or until thickened. Makes 3 servings.

Calories: 95 *Fat: 0.8 gram*
Protein: 6 grams *Fibre: 4.5 grams*
Carbohydrates: 19 grams
Sodium: 349 milligrams

Steamed Fresh Vegetables

Large-Volume Recipe

1 pound baby carrots
4 medium courgettes, cut in 2-inch chunks
2 pounds broccoli florets
1 pound asparagus, trimmed
8 ounces mushrooms, stems removed

In a very large pot, place a steamer basket and 1 inch of water. In order, add carrots, courgettes, broccoli, asparagus, and mushrooms to the pot. Steam on high heat for 8 to 10 minutes until asparagus is crisp-tender. Makes 8 servings.

Calories: 79 *Fat: 1 gram*
Protein: 6 grams *Fibre: 6 grams*
Carbohydrates: 16 grams
Sodium: 48 milligrams

Broccoli Mushroom Sauté

Quick

1 pound broccoli florets
2 ounces thinly sliced spring onions
4 garlic cloves, minced
8 ounces mushrooms, sliced
2 tablespoons lemon juice
½ teaspoon salt
¼ teaspoon pepper

In a large pot, bring 1 inch of water to a boil. Place broccoli in a steamer basket over the water; cover pot and steam for 4 to 5 minutes or until crisp-tender. In a pan coated with non-stick cooking spray, sauté onions over medium heat for 2 minutes. Add garlic and mushrooms and cook for 2 minutes. Add the cooked broccoli, the lemon juice, salt, and pepper; toss to coat. Remove from heat and serve. Makes 6 servings.

Calories: 31 *Fat: 0.3 gram*
Protein: 3 grams *Fibre: 2.6 grams*
Carbohydrates: 6 grams
Sodium: 214 milligrams

SNACKS AND APPETIZERS

Salmon Crackers

1 tablespoon salsa
1 ounce canned salmon, drained
1 ounce non-fat cream cheese
2 fat-free Ry-Krisp crackers

Mix salsa with salmon. Place half of cream cheese and salmon mix on each cracker. Makes 1 serving.

Calories: 116 *Fat: 2 grams*
Protein: 12 grams *Fibre: 4 grams*
Carbohydrates: 12 grams
Sodium: 433 milligrams

Cottage Cheese and Yogurt Mix

2 ounces non-fat cottage cheese
4 ounces non-fat yogurt (unsweetened, or sweetened with sugar substitute)

Mix together cottage cheese and yogurt for a great snack. Makes 1 serving.

Calories: 121 *Fat: 0 gram*
Protein: 19 grams *Fibre: 0 gram*
Carbohydrates: 10 grams
Sodium: 370 milligrams

Black Bean Pinwheels

8 ounces non-fat cream cheese
8 ounces non-fat sour cream
4 ounces non-fat shredded Cheddar cheese
¼ teaspoon garlic powder
One 15-ounce can black beans, drained
Ten 10-inch whole-wheat flour tortillas
Salsa

Blend cream cheese and sour cream in a medium bowl. Stir in cheese and garlic powder. Cover and refrigerate for 2 hours. Process beans in a food processor until smooth. Spread a thin layer of the beans and then a thin layer of the cheese mixture over each tortilla. Roll each tortilla up tightly. Wrap in plastic wrap and refrigerate until chilled. Cut each tortilla crosswise into 7 slices. Serve with salsa. Makes about 24 servings (3 slices per serving).

Calories: 120 *Fat: 1 gram*
Protein: 9 grams *Fibre: 2.6 grams*
Carbohydrates: 21 grams
Sodium: 504 milligrams

Beans and Salsa Dip

Quick and Large-Volume Recipe

6 fl. ounces salsa
3 ½ ounces non-fat refried beans
3 ounces black beans

Mix all the ingredients together. Serve with baked tortilla chips or vegetables. Makes 8 servings (4 tablespoons per serving).

Calories: 36 grams *Fat: 0 gram*
Protein: 2 grams *Fibre: 2 grams*
Carbohydrates: 6 grams
Sodium: 208 milligrams

Chicken Stuffed Potato

Quick

1 medium baking potato
3 ounces cooked chicken breast, chopped
2 tablespoons salsa

Use a fork and pierce the potato skin. Bake the potato in a microwave on high for 7 to 10 minutes or until tender. Slice open and fill with chicken. Top with salsa. Makes 1 serving.

Calories: 368 *Fat: 3 grams*
Protein: 31 grams *Fibre: 5 grams*
Carbohydrates: 52 grams
Sodium: 631 milligrams

Baked Potato Topped with Cottage Cheese

Quick

1 medium baking potato
4 ounces non-fat cottage cheese
Salsa (optional)

Use a fork and pierce the potato skin. Bake the potato in a microwave on high for 7 to 10 minutes or until tender. Slice open and fill with cottage cheese. Top with salsa. Makes 1 serving.

Calories: 342 *Fat: 0 gram*
Protein: 29 grams *Fibre: 5 grams*
Carbohydrates: 54 grams
Sodium: 597 milligrams

Cowboy Caviar

by Jan Lutz

Quick and Large-Volume Recipe

Great for BBQs or potlucks!
Two 15-ounce cans black beans, rinsed and drained
10-ounce bag frozen white corn, thawed
1 pint cherry tomatoes, diced
1 medium red onion, diced
½ bunch cilantro, chopped
2 ripe avocados, diced

Combine all ingredients. Serve as a dip. Makes 20 servings.

Calories: 110 *Fat: 3.5 grams*
Protein: 5 grams *Fibre: 5.5 grams*
Carbohydrates: 17 grams
Sodium: 105 milligrams

Tuna Spread for Whatever

by Nancy Van Hoven

Quick

6 ounces albacore tuna, drained
6 egg whites, cooked
1 tablespoon chopped green onion
2 tablespoons chopped celery
2 fl. ounces fat-free Thousand Island dressing

Mix all ingredients together. Serve on rye crackers, pitta bread, stuff into tomatoes, use as a vegetable dip, or whatever! Makes 4 servings.

Calories: 97 *Fat: 0.7 grams*
Protein: 16 grams *Fibre: 0 gram*
Carbohydrates: 7 grams
Sodium: 480 milligrams

Blueberry–Peach Smoothie

Quick

8 ounces non-fat vanilla yogurt
5 ounces fresh blueberries
1 medium peach, sliced
Ice

Blend all the ingredients together, adding the ice cubes a few at a time until shake is the desired consistency. Makes 1 serving.

Calories: 208 *Fat: 0.6 gram*
Protein: 15 grams *Fibre: 5 grams*
Carbohydrates: 39
Sodium: 161 milligrams

Banana–Strawberry Smoothie

Quick

8 ounces non-fat vanilla yogurt
5 ounces fresh strawberry halves
1 medium banana, sliced
2 fl. ounces apple juice
Ice

Blend all the ingredients together, adding the ice cubes a few at a time until shake is the desired consistency. Makes 1 serving.

Calories: 274 *Fat: 1 gram*
Protein: 15 grams *Fibre: 7 grams*
Carbohydrates: 56 grams
Sodium: 163 milligrams

Fat-Free Cinnamon Rolls

Large-Volume Recipe

Dough

6 fl. ounces non-fat milk
3½ ounces sugar
1 teaspoon salt
6 ounces unsweetened apple-sauce
2 packets active dry yeast
3 fl. ounces warm water
4 egg whites
12½ ounces whole-wheat flour
12½ ounces all-purpose flour

Filling

3 tablespoons light margarine
2 teaspoons ground cinnamon
3½ ounces brown sugar
1 ¾ ounces granulated sugar

Glaze/Topping

3 fl. ounces evaporated skimmed milk
2 tablespoons packed brown sugar
7½ ounces icing sugar
1 teaspoon vanilla flavouring

To make the dough, combine milk, sugar, salt, and applesauce in a bowl. Microwave for 1 to 2 minutes until sugar dissolves. Cool to lukewarm. Dissolve yeast in warm water. Add milk mixture, egg whites, and 2 cups of *each* of the flours. Attach dough hook to electric heavy-duty mixer. Turn to low-medium speed and mix for 2 minutes or knead by hand. Continue on low-medium speed, adding remaining flour, 2½ ounces at a time, until dough clings to hook and side of the bowl, about 2 minutes. Continue kneading for another 2 minutes. Place dough in greased bowl, turning it over to grease entire surface. Cover; let rise in warm place, free from drafts, until doubled in bulk, about 1 hour. Punch down dough. Place dough on floured surface and roll out to ¼-inch thick. Spread light margarine lightly over surface. Sprinkle with brown sugar, cinnamon, and very lightly with granulated sugar. Roll up dough from long side. Slice rolled dough using a serrated knife into 21 rolls and place on greased baking sheet. Let rise for 45 to 60 minutes. Preheat oven to 350°F/180°C/GM4. Bake for 15 to 18 minutes until light brown in colour. Let rolls cool in pan.

For glaze, heat milk and brown sugar in microwave for 1 minute or until brown sugar dissolves. Whip in icing sugar and vanilla until creamy. Pour over rolls. Store in sealed container. Makes 21 servings.

Each roll:
Calories: 201 *Fat: 0.5 grams*
Protein: 5 grams *Fibre: 2 grams*
Carbohydrates: 45 grams
Sodium: 160 milligrams

Maple Bars

Large-Volume Recipe

Dough for Fat-Free Cinnamon Rolls (page 209)

Glaze
3 fl. ounces evaporated skimmed milk
2 tablespoons packed brown sugar
7½ ounces icing sugar
½ teaspoon maple extract

Follow the directions for the cinnamon rolls until you roll out the dough. For these bars, place the dough on a floured surface and roll it out to about 1-inch thick. Cut into 16 rectangles. Place on greased baking sheet and let rise for 40 minutes. Preheat oven to 350°F/180°C/GM4. Bake for 15 to 22 minutes or until lightly brown. Make the glaze in the same manner as for the cinnamon roll glaze. Makes 16 servings.

Calories: 250 *Fat: 0.6 gram*
Protein: 7 grams *Fibre: 2.6 grams*
Carbohydrates: 53 grams
Sodium: 200 milligrams

Whole-Wheat Banana Bread

5 ounces flour
3 3/4 ounces whole-wheat flour
1 teaspoon baking soda
1/4 teaspoon salt
1/2 cup sugar
3/4 cup unsweetened applesauce
2 egg whites
2 ripe bananas, mashed
1 teaspoon pure vanilla

Preheat oven to 350°F/180°C/GM4. Spray a 1 1/2 quart loaf pan with non-stick cooking spray. Mix all dry ingredients in a medium bowl. Beat all other ingredients in a large bowl. Slowly add flour mixture to applesauce mixture and mix well. Pour into prepared pan. Bake for 40 to 45 minutes until toothpick inserted in centre of loaf comes out clean. Makes 12 servings.

Calories: 123 *Fat: 0.3 gram*
Protein: 3 grams *Fibre: 2 grams*
Carbohydrates: 28 grams
Sodium: 161 milligrams

Fruit Pizza

Large-Volume Recipe

One 18-ounce roll shop-bought sugar cookie dough
2 1/2 ounces whole-wheat flour
One 8-ounce package non-fat cream cheese
5 ounces icing sugar
1/4 teaspoon almond extract
5 1/2 ounces apricot jam
3 large kiwis, sliced
10 ounces sliced strawberries
1 small can pineapple chunks, drained

Preheat oven to 350°F/180°C/GM4s. Roll out cookie dough on whole-wheat floured surface. Make a 16-inch circle with dough. Bake on a baking sheet for 15 minutes. Let cool. Mix cream cheese, icing sugar, and almond extract until creamy. Spread cream cheese mixture over baked cookie crust. On top of cream cheese mixture, spread the apricot jam to make a thin layer. Arrange fruit on top of pizza as you like. Refrigerate for 1 to 2 hours. Makes 16 servings.

Calories: 235 *Fat: 7 grams*
Protein: 8 grams *Fibre: 2 grams*
Carbohydrates: 35 grams
Sodium: 371 milligrams

Low-fat Creamy Cheesecake

10 low-fat digestives
Three 8-ounce packages non-fat cream cheese
16 ounces non-fat sour cream
3 egg whites
5¼ ounces sugar (or sugar substitute)
¾ teaspoon salt (optional)
¼ teaspoon ground ginger
2 teaspoon pure vanilla flavouring

Preheat oven to 350°F/180°C/GM4. Crush graham crackers and line bottom of 9-inch springform pan with them. Whip cream cheese until smooth. Add sour cream and blend until smooth. Add the remaining ingredients. Pour mixture over crushed graham crackers in pan. Bake for 52 to 60 minutes until middle of cheese-cake does not jiggle. Cool in pan. Cover and chill for at least 2 hours or overnight. Makes 8 servings.

Optional: For toppings, add your favourite fruit such as sliced strawberries, raspberries, blueberries, or cooked apples.

Calories: 241 *Fat: 2 grams*
Protein: 16 grams *Fibre: 1 gram*
Carbohydrates: 38 grams
Sodium: 600 milligrams

Banana Cream Dessert

Two 2.1-ounce packages fat-free, sugar-free vanilla custard mix
1 pint non-fat milk
2 fl. ounces fat-free vanilla coffee creamer
10 low-fat graham crackers, crushed
1 medium banana
Non-fat whipped cream

Prepare mix as directed on package except add milk and vanilla coffee creamer. Line a 9-inch glass pie plate with graham cracker crumbs. Slice one-half of the banana and arrange on top of the cracker crumbs. Pour pudding mix over bananas. Slice the other one-half of the banana and arrange on top. Top with non-fat whipped cream and refrigerate for 2 hours. Makes 8 servings.

Calories: 203 *Fat: 3.5 grams*
Protein: 5 grams *Fibre: 1 gram*
Carbohydrates: 37 grams
Sodium: 831 milligrams

Oatmeal Raisin Cookies

Large-Volume Recipe

12 ounces unsweetened applesauce
5¼ ounces packed brown sugar
3½ ounces granulated sugar (or sugar substitute)
4 egg whites
1 teaspoon pure vanilla flavouring
3¾ ounces all-purpose flour
3¾ ounces whole-wheat flour
1 teaspoon baking soda
1 teaspoon ground cinnamon
½ teaspoon salt (optional)
4 ounces vanilla protein powder
9 ounces porridge oats, uncooked
5 ounces raisins

Preheat oven to 350°F/180°C/GM4. Beat applesauce and sugars together. Add egg whites and vanilla; beat well. In separate bowl, combine flours, baking soda, cinnamon, salt, and protein powder. Add slowly to applesauce mixture until blended. Add oats and raisins. Drop by teaspoons on baking sheet and bake for 14 minutes. Cookies will be soft in middle, but not gooey. Cool on wire rack. Makes 3 dozen.

Calories: 83 *Fat: 0.2 gram*
Protein: 2 grams *Fibre: 2 grams*
Carbohydrates: 19 grams
Sodium: 46 milligrams

Sugar-Free Oatmeal Cookies

by Cindy Marshall

3½ ounces sugar substitute
1 small package sugar-free instant banana custard mix
6¼ ounces whole-wheat flour
1 teaspoon baking soda
1 teaspoon salt
7½ ounces uncooked porridge oats
1 teaspoon ground cinnamon
1 teaspoon ground nutmeg
1½ ounces chopped pecans
8 ounces light vanilla yogurt
4 egg whites
2 fl. ounces non-fat milk
2 teaspoons vanilla
5 ounces raisins

Preheat oven to 350°F/180°C/GM4. Spray cooking sheet with non-stick cooking spray. Mix dry ingredients together. Add remaining ingredients. Mix well. Spoon dough onto prepared pan, spacing spoonfuls one inch apart. Press slightly to flatten. Bake for 10 to 12 minutes. Cookies will be soft in middle, but not gooey. Makes 2 dozen.

Calories: 90 *Fat: 1.5 grams*
Protein: 3 grams *Fibre: 2 grams*
Carbohydrates: 17 grams
Sodium: 130 milligrams

Whole-Wheat Chocolate Chip Cookies

6¼ cups all-purpose flour
5 ounces whole-wheat flour
1 teaspoon baking soda
¾ teaspoon salt (optional)
12 ounces unsweetened applesauce
5¼ ounces granulated sugar
5¼ ounces packed brown sugar
1 teaspoon vanilla
4 egg whites
6 ounces dark chocolate chips
2 ounces chopped walnuts (optional)

Preheat oven to 375°F/190°C/GM5. Combine flours, baking soda, and salt in a small bowl. Beat applesauce, sugars, and vanilla in a large mixing bowl. Add egg whites and beat well. Gradually add flour mixture. Stir in chocolate chips and nuts. Drop the dough by teaspoons one inch apart onto a baking sheet. Bake for 10 to 13 minutes or until golden brown. Makes 4 dozen cookies.

Calories: 75 *Fat: 2 grams*
Protein: 1 gram *Fibre: 1 gram*
Carbohydrates: 14 grams
Sodium: 69 milligrams

Baked Apple

1 baking apple (Golden Delicious, Jonathan)
1 tablespoon apple juice
½ teaspoon sugar substitute
½ teaspoon ground cinnamon

Preheat oven to 350°F/180°C/GM4. Remove the stem and core of apple, making a hole all the way through. Place in a glass baking dish. Pour apple juice over the apple, then sprinkle with sugar substitute and cinnamon. Bake, uncovered, for 45 minutes. Or cover with plastic wrap and microwave for 7 to 10 minutes or until apple is tender. Makes 1 serving.

Calories: 82 *Fat: 0.5 grams*
Protein: 1 gram *Fibre: 5 grams*
Carbohydrates: 21 grams
Sodium: 3 milligrams

Mock Apple Pie

2 ounces porridge oats, uncooked
7 cooking apples (Golden Delicious, Rome, Granny Smith)
3½ ounces sugar substitute
1 tablespoon ground cinnamon
4 fl. ounces apple juice
1 tablespoon whole-wheat flour
4 ounces vanilla protein powder

Preheat oven to 350°F/180°C/GM4. Spray 9-inch pie pan with non-stick spray. Sprinkle ⅓ of the oats in bottom. Slice or shred apple (cored) with peel and place in large mixing bowl. Add sugar substitute, cinnamon, apple juice, and flour. Pour into pie pan. Mix remaining oats with protein powder. Pour over apples. Spray topping with cooking spray to provide moisture. Bake for 35 minutes uncovered, and then cover with foil and bake for 10 more minutes. Makes 12 servings.

Calories: 153 *Fat: 2 grams*
Protein: 5 grams *Fibre: 5 grams*
Carbohydrates: 31 grams
Sodium: 82 milligrams

APPLE VARIETIES

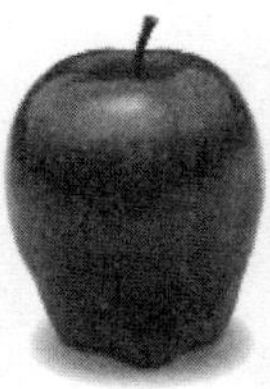

Red Delicious
Deep ruby skin and a classic heart shape. Its mild, sweet flavour and juicy crunch make it one of the most popular snacking apples

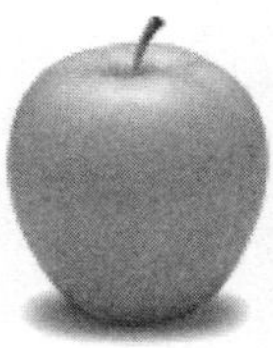

Golden Delicious
The preferred all-purpose cooking apple. Firm, white flesh and skin so tender it doesn't require peeling. Maintains its shape and rich, mellow flavour after cooking.

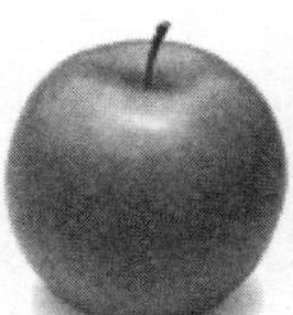

Granny Smith
Bright green, sometimes with a pink blush. Tart, tangy flavour and crisp bite. Great for cooking or as a take-along snack.

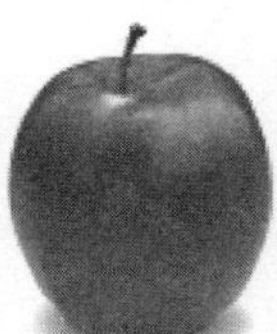

Pink Lady
Delicious sweet-tart taste and firm, crisp flesh. Yellow in colour with a pink blush. A great apple for cooking or eating out of hand.

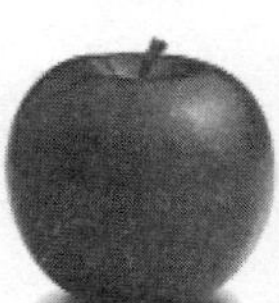

Rome Beauty
Bright red, used primarily for cooking because the flavour grows richer when the apple is baked or sautéed. Often referred to as the "baker's buddy".

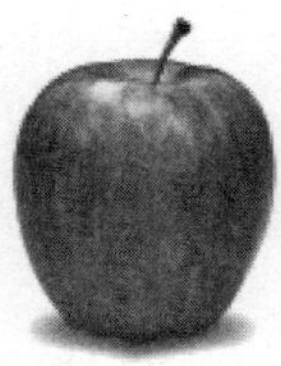

Gala
Heart shaped, distinctive yellow-orange skin with red striping and a crisp, sweet taste. Great in salads or eating out of hand.

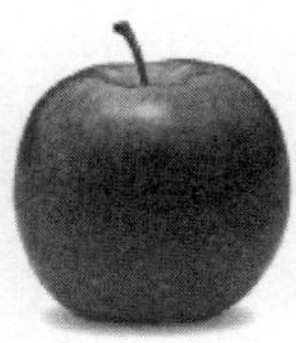

Fuji
Varies from yellow-green with red highlights to very red. Crisp and juicy with a spicy, sweet flavour. Excellent in salads or eating out of hand.

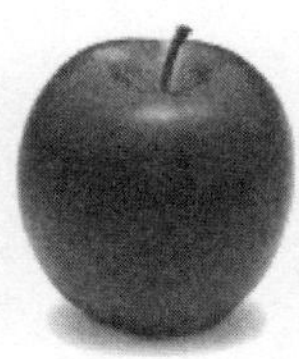

Braeburn
Varying from greenish gold with red sections to nearly solid red, its crisp, aromatic blend of sweetness and tartness delivers high-impact flavour. Great for snacks or salads.

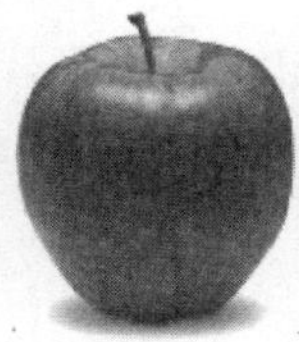

Cameo
Offers rich, sweet taste and firm texture. It has a red stripe over a creamy background. Excellent for desserts or snacking.

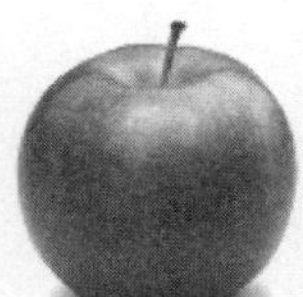

Jonagold
A blend of Jonathan and Golden Delicious. Yellow-green base with a blush stripe. Unique tangy-sweet flavour. Great for cooking or just plain eating.

APPENDIX

Food and Beverage Record

Date From____________ to____________

Day____________________

Time	Food/Beverage and Quantity	Calories	Protein (g)	Carbs (g)	Fat (g)	Fibre (g)
	Totals:					

Weekly Exercise Tracking

Week #_____

Day/Date	**Cardiovascular**	**Intensity (heart rate*)**	**Duration (minutes)**	**Weight Training**	**Comments**
Monday _____	__Treadmill __Bike __Stair step __Aerobic class _________Other	__80–100 __110–130 __140–160 __160–180	__10–20 __25–35 __40–60 __60–90	__Upper body __Lower body __Overall body __Sculpt or group class	
Tuesday _____	__Treadmill __Bike __Stair step __Aerobic class _________Other	__80–100 __110–130 __140–160 __160–180	__10–20 __25–35 __40–60 __60–90	__Upper body __Lower body __Overall __Sculpt or group class	
Wednesday _____	__Treadmill __Bike __Stair step __Aerobic class _________Other	__80–100 __110–130 __140–160 __160–180	__10–20 __25–35 __40–60 __60–90	__Upper body __Lower body __Overall __Sculpt or group class	
Thursday _____	__Treadmill __Bike __Stair step __Aerobic class _________Other	__80–100 __110–130 __140–160 __160–180	__10–20 __25–35 __40–60 __60–90	__Upper body __Lower body __Overall __Sculpt or group class	

Friday _____	__Treadmill __Stair step _________Other	__Bike __Aerobic class	__80–100 __140–160	__110–130 __160–180	__10–20 __40–60	__25–35 __60–90	__Upper body __Lower body __Overall __Sculpt or group class	
Saturday _____	__Treadmill __Stair step _________Other	__Bike __Aerobic class	__80–100 __140–160	__110–130 __160–180	__10–20 __40–60	__25–35 __60–90	__Upper body __Lower body __Overall __Sculpt or group class	
Sunday _____	__Treadmill __Stair step _________Other	__Bike __Aerobic class	__80–100 __140–160	__110–130 __160–180	__10–20 __40–60	__25–35 __60–90	__Upper body __Lower body __Overall __Sculpt or group class	
Sample *1/15/03*	__Treadmill __Stair step _________Other	X Bike __Aerobic class	__80–100 X 140–160	__110–130 __160–180	__10–20 X 40–60	__25–35 __60–90	__Upper body __Lower body X Overall __Sculpt or group class	Exercise felt great

*To find your heart rate, wear a heart rate monitor or check your pulse on the wrist or neck. Count the beats over 6 seconds then multiply the number by 10. For example: The number of beats after 6 seconds is 13; 13 × 10 = 130 beats per minute.

Target heart rate calculation: 220 − age = maximum heart rate. Take your maximum heart rate and multiply it by 65 per cent and then 85 per cent to get your target heart rate range. Example: 220 − 36 = 184; 184 × 0.65 = 120 beats per minute; 184 × 0.85 = 156 beats per minute. Your target is 120 to 156 beats per minute.

BEFORE PHOTOS

Place "before" photo here.
—FRONT—

Place "before" photo here.
—BACK—

AFTER PHOTOS

Place "after" photo here.
—FRONT—

Place "after" photo here.
—BACK—

BEFORE PHOTOS

Place "before" photo here.
—FRONT—

Place "before" photo here.
—BACK—

AFTER PHOTOS

Place "after" photo here.
—FRONT—

Place "after" photo here.
—BACK—

BIBLIOGRAPHY

American Dietetic Association. "Dietary Reference Intakes Released for Carbohydrates, Fats, Protein, fibre and Physical Activity." *Dietetics in Practice*, Fall 2002; volume 2, Chicago, IL.

American Heart Association. "Media Advisory: American Heart Association's Statement on High-Protein, Low-Carbohydrate Diet Study." Paper presented at Scientific Sessions. Nov 2002.

Barzel US, Massey LK. "Excess dietary protein can adversely affect bone." *J Nutr* 1998;128:1051–53.

Bessesen DH. "The role of carbohydrates in insulin resistance". *J Nutr* 2001;131:2782S.

Brand-Miller J, Wolever T, Colagiuri S, and Foster-Powell K. *The Glucose Revolution*. Marlowe, New York, 1999.

———. *The New Glucose Revolution*. Marlowe, New York, 2003.

Clark N. *Sports Nutrition Guidebook*. Human Kinetics, Champaign IL, 1997.

Conceicao de Oliveira M, Sichieri R, and Moura AS. "Weight loss associated with a daily intake of three apples or three pears among overweight women." *Nutr* 2003;19:253–56.

Davy BM, and Melby CL. "The effect of fibre-rich carbohydrates on features of Syndrome X." *J Am Diet Assoc* 2003;103:86–96.

DesMaisons K. *Potatoes not Prozac*. Simon & Schuster, New York, 1998.

Evans W, and Rosenberg I. *BioMarkers*. Simon & Schuster, New York, 1992.

Foster-Powell K, and Miller JB. "International tables of glycemic index." *Am J Clin Nutr* 1995;62:871S.

Freese R, Alfthan G, Jauhiainen M, et al. "High intakes of vegetables, berries, and apples combined with a high intake of linoleic or oleic acid only slightly affect markers of lipid peroxidation and lipoprotein metabolism in healthy subjects." *Am J Clin Nutr* 2002;76:950–60.

Frost G, Lees A, Dore CJ, et al. "Glycemic index as a determinant of serum HDL-cholesterol concentration." *Lancet* 1999;353:1045.

Golay A, Eigenheer C, Morel Y, et al. "Weight loss with low or high carbohydrate diet?" *Int J Obes Relat Metab Disord* 1996;20:1067.

Heshka S, Yang MU, Wang J, et al. "Weight loss and changes in resting metabolic rate." *Am J Clin Nutr* 1990;52:981–86.

Hill JO, Melanson EL, and Wyatt HT. "Dietary fat intake and regulation of energy balance: Implications for obesity." *J Nutr* 2000;130: 284S–288S.

Howarth NC, Saltzman E, and Roberts SB. "Dietary fibre and weight regulation." *Nutr Rev* 2001;59:129.

Hyson D, Studebarker-Hallman D, Davis PA, et al. "Apple juice consumption reduces plasma Low-Density Lipoprotein oxidation in healthy men and women." *J of Med Food* 2000;3:159–65.

Insel P, Turner RE, and Ross D. *Nutrition*. Jones & Bartlett, Sudbury, MA 2001.

Jenkins DJ, Wolever TM, Vuksan V, et al. "Nibbling versus gorging: metabolic advantages of increased meal frequency." *New Eng J Med* 1989;321:929–34.

Jequier E. "Response to and range of acceptable fat intake in adults." *Eur J Clin Nutr* 1999; 53:S84–93.

Katan MB. "Are there good and bad carbohydrates for HDL cholesterol?" *Lancet* 1999;353:1029.

Katz D. *The Way to Eat*. Sourcebooks, Naperville, IL 2002.

Keim NL, Van Loan MD, Horn WF, et al. "Weight loss is greater with consumption of large morning meals and fat-free mass is preserved with large evening meals in women on a controlled weight reduction regimen." *J Nutr* 1997;127:75–82.

Kelsay JL, Behall KM, and Prather ES. "Effect of fibre from fruits and vegetables on metabolic responses of human subjects I. Bowel transit time, number of defecations, fecal weight, urinary excretions of energy and nitrogen and apparent digestibilities of energy, nitrogen, and fat." *Am J Clin Nutr* 1978;31:1149–53.

Klem ML, Wing RR, McGuire MT, et al. "A descriptive study of individuals successful at long-term maintenance of substantial weight loss." *Am J Clin Nutr* 1997;66:239–46.

Lampe JA. "Health effects of vegetables and fruit: assessing mechanisms of action in human experimental studies." *Am J Clin Nutr* 1999;70:475S–490S

Layman DK, Boileau RA, Erickson D et al. "A reduced ratio of dietary carbohydrates to protein improves body composition and blood lipid profiles during weight loss in adult women." *J Nutr* 2003;133:411–17.

Layman DK, Shiue H, Sather C. et al. "Increased dietary protein modifies glucose and insulin homeostasis in adult women during weight loss." *J Nutr* 2003;133:405–10.

Levine AS, and Billington CJ. "Dietary fibre: does it affect food intake and body weight?" In Fernstrom JD and Miller GD, editors, *Appetite and Body Weight Regulation: Sugar, Fat, and Macronutrient Substitutes*. CRC Press, Boca Raton, FL, 1994:191–200.

Ludwig DS, Majzoub JA, et al. "High glycemic-index foods, overeating, and obesity." *Pediatrics* 1999; Vol. 103, No. 3, 103–26.

McCrory MA, Fuss PJ, Saltzman E, et al. "Dietary determinants of energy intake and weight regulation in healthy adults." *J Nutr* 2000;130:276S.

Mayo Clinic. "Special Report: Weight Control." Supplement to Foundation for Medical Education and Research Publications, Rochester, MN, 2003.

Moore MC, Cherrington AD, Mann SL, et al. "Acute fructose administration decreases the glycemic response to an oral glucose tolerance test in normal adults." *Clin Endocrinol Metab* 2000;85:4515.

Muldoon MF, and Kritchevsky SB. "Flavonoid intake and coronary mortality in Finland: a cohort study." *Br Med J* 1996;312:478–81.

Raben A, Christensen NJ, Madsen J, et al. "Decreased postprandial thermogenesis and fat oxidation but increased fullness after a high-fibre meal compared with a low-fibre meal." *Am J Clin Nutr* 1994;59: 1386–94.

Roberts SB. "High-glycemic index foods, hunger, and obesity: is there a connection?" *Nutr Rev* 2000;58:163.

Rolls B. "The role of energy density in the overconsumption of fat." *J Nutr* 2000;130:268S–271S.

Rolls B, Bell EA, Castellanos VH, et al. "Energy density but not fat content of foods affected energy intake in lean and obese women." *Am J Clin Nutr* 1999 May;69:863–71.

Simopoulos AP. "Essential fatty acids in health and chronic disease." *Am J Clin Nutr* 1999; 70:560S–569S.

Simopoulos AP, and Robinson J. *The Omega Diet*. Harper Perennial, New York, 1999.

Wing RR, and Hill JO. "Successful weight loss maintenance." *Annu Rev Nutr* 2001;21:323–41.

Resources and Recommended Reading

American Academy of Family Physicians	**www.aafp.org**
American Diabetes Association	**www.diabetes.org**
American Dietetic Association	**www.eatright.org**
American Medical Association	**www.ama-assn.org**
Centers for Disease Control and Prevention	**www.cdc.gov**
U.S. Department of Agriculture: Food and Nutrition Information Center	**www.nal.usda.gov/fnic**
Weight Control Information Network	**www.niddk.nih.gov/health/nutrit/win.htm**

- *Body for Life* by Bill Phillips.
- *Food Values of Portions Commonly Used* by Jean A. T. Pennington.
- *Food Works* nutrition analysis software.
- *New Cook Book* by Better Homes and Gardens.
- *Sports Nutrition Guidebook* by Nancy Clark.
- *The NutriBase Complete Book of Food Counts,* Nutribase.
- *Women's Health & Wellness 2003: Real-Life Solutions from the Editors of* Health *Magazine.*

RECIPE INDEX

Breakfast Foods

Protein Foods

EGGS

SHAKES

CHICKEN, TURKEY, FISH, AND BEEF

Combination Foods

MAIN ENTRÉES

Salads and Vegetables

Snacks and Appetizers

Desserts and Sweets

INDEX